Preimplantation Mammalian Embryos In Vitro: Recent Studies. I.

Papers by
Shuetu Suzuki, Benjamin G. Brackett,
T. Iwamatsu, M. C. Chang, H. M. Seitz,
Richard Stambaugh, Stella Pickworth,
Antonin Pavlok, R. Yanagimachi, Ralph
Brinster, K. A. O. Ellem, Richard J.
Tasca, R. G. Wales, Joan L. Thomson,
Susan Auerbach, J. C. Daniel, Cole
Manes, et al.

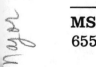

15.⁰⁰

12-1-72

Major

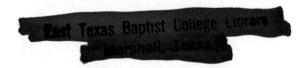
MSS Information Corporation
655 Madison Avenue, New York, N.Y. 10021

Library of Congress Cataloging in Publication Data
Main entry under title:

Preimplantation mammalian embryos in vitro.

   Includes bibliographies.
   1. Embryology--Mammals--Addresses, essays, lectures.
2. Fertilization (Biology)--Addresses, essays, lectures.
I. Suzuki, Shuetu. [DNLM: 1. Mammals--Embryology--
Collected works. 2. Nidation--Collected works.
QS 645 P924]
QL959.P7   599'.03'3   72-6668
ISBN 0-8422-7039-6

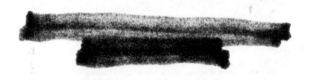

TABLE OF CONTENTS

CREDITS & ACKNOWLEDGEMENTS

Auerbach, Susan; and R. L. Brinster, "Lactate Dehydrogenase Isozymes in Mouse Blastocyst Cultures," *Experimental Cell Research*, 1968, 53:313-315.

Auerbach, Susan; and R. L. Brinster, "Lactate Dehydrogenase Isozymes in the Early Mouse Embryo," *Experimental Cell Research*, 1967, 46:89-92.

Brackett, Benjamin G., "Effects of Washing the Gametes on Fertilization *In Vitro*," *Fertility and Sterility*, 1969, 20:127-142.

Brackett, Benjamin G., "*In Vitro* Fertilization of Rabbit Ova: Time Sequence of Events," *Fertility and Sterility*, 1970, 21:169-176.

Brackett, Benjamin G.; and William L. Williams, "Fertilization of Rabbit Ova in a Defined Medium," *Fertility and Sterility*, 1968, 19:144-155.

Brinster, R. L., "Incorporation of Carbon from Glucose and Pyruvate into the Preimplantation Mouse Embryo," *Experimental Cell Research*, 1969, 58:153-158.

Brinster, R. L., "Radioactive Carbon Dioxide Production from Pyruvate and Lactate by the Preimplantation Rabbit Embryo," *Experimental Cell Research*, 1969, 54:205-209.

Chang, M. C., "*In Vitro* Fertilization of Mammalian Eggs," *Journal of Animal Science*, 1968, 27(Suppl. 1): 15-22.

Daniel, J. C., Jr., "The Pattern of Utilization of Respiratory Metabolic Intermediates by Preimplantation Rabbit Embryos *in Vitro*," *Experimental Cell Research*, 1967, 47:619-624.

Ellem, K. A. O.; and R. B. L. Gwatkin, "Patterns of Nucleic Acid Synthesis in the Early Mouse Embryo," *Developmental Biology*, 1968, 18:311-330.

Iwamatsu, T.; and M. C. Chang, "*In vitro* Fertilization of Mouse Eggs in the Presence of Bovine Follicular Fluid," *Nature*, 1969, 224:919-920.

Manes, Cole, "Nucleic Acid Synthesis in Preimplantation Rabbit Embryos. I. Quantitative Aspects, Relationship to Early Morphogenesis and Protein Synthesis," *The Journal of Experimental Zoology*, 1969, 172:303-310.

Manes, Cole, "Nucleic Acid Synthesis in Preimplantation Rabbit Embryos. II. Delayed Synthesis of Ribosomal RNA," *The Journal of Experimental Zoology*, 1971, 176:87-96.

Manes, Cole; and J. C. Daniel, Jr., "Quantitative and Qualitative Aspects of Protein Synthesis in the Preimplantation Rabbit Embryo," *Experimental Cell Research*, 1969, 55:261-268.

Pavlok, Antonin, "Fertilization of Mouse Ova *in Vitro*. I. Effect of Some Factors on Fertilization," *Journal of Reproductive Fertility*, 1968, 16:401-408.

Pickworth, Stella; and M. C. Chang, "Fertilization of Chinese Hamster Eggs *in Vitro*," *Journal of Reproductive Fertility*, 1969, 19:371-374.

Seitz, H. M., Jr.; Benjamin G. Brackett; and Luigi Mastroianni, Jr., "*In Vitro* Fertilization of Ovulated Rabbit Ova Recovered from the Ovary," *Biology of Reproduction*, 1970, 2:262-267.

Stambaugh, Richard; Benjamin G. Brackett; and Luigi Mastroianni, "Inhibition of *in Vitro* Fertilization of Rabbit Ova by Trypsin Inhibitors," *Biology of Reproduction*, 1969, 1:223-227.

Suzuki, Shuetu; and Luigi Mastroianni, Jr., "*In-Vitro* Fertilization of Rabbit Follicular Oocytes in Tubal Fluid," *Fertility and Sterility*, 1968, 19:716-725.

Tasca, Richard J.; and Nina Hillman, "Effects of Actinomycin D and Cycloheximide on RNA and Protein Synthesis in Cleavage Stage Mouse Embryos," *Nature*, 1970, 225:1022-1025.

TenBroeck, Joan Thompson, "Effect of Nucleosides and Nucleoside Bases on the Development of Pre-implantation Mouse Embryos *in Vitro*," *Journal of Reproductive Fertility*, 1968, 17:571-573.

Thompson, Joan L.; and Ralph L. Brinster, "Glycogen Content of Preimplantation Mouse Embryos," *The Anatomical Record*, 1966, 155:97-102.

Wales, R. G.; and J. D. Biggers, "The Permeability of Two- and Eight-cell Mouse Embryos to L-Malic Acid," *Journal of Reproductive Fertility*, 1968, 15:103-111.

Wales, R. G.; and R. L. Brinster, "The Uptake of Hexoses by Pre-implantation Mouse Embryos *in Vitro*," *Journal of Reproductive Fertility*, 1968, 15:415-422.

Wales, R. G.; P. Quinn; and R. N. Murdoch, "The Fixation of Carbon Dioxide by the Eight-cell Mouse Embryo," *Journal of Reproductive Fertility*, 1969, 20:541-543.

Yanagimachi, R.; and Y. D. Noda, "Physiological Changes in the Postnuclear Cap Region of Mammalian Spermatozoa: A Necessary Preliminary to the Membrane Fusion between Sperm and Egg Cells," *Journal of Ultrastructure Research*, 1970, 31:486-493.

PREFACE

The recent development of a technology permitting growth of preimplantation mammalian embryos *in vitro* has made it possible for scientists to investigate experimentally the early events of mammalian embryogenesis. The growing volume of experimental work based on these new *in vitro* techniques permits, for the first time, a more penetrating description of the early stages of mammalian life. Prior to this, study of mammalian embryos was largely confined to morphological observations.

The present two-volume collection includes papers published during the period 1968-1971 which deal with the fertilization of mammalian eggs *in vitro* and describe the development of these eggs up to the blastocyst stage. Investigations concerning the molecular biology and other biochemical attributes of early mammalian development are presented in these volumes, though in this area studies with mammalian material are only now approaching a high level of sophistication, due mainly to the formidable technical problems arising from the relatively minute amounts of experimental material available. Also included in this collection are papers describing a variety of elegant micromanipulation experiments with mammalian eggs, particularly experiments in which chimaeric embryos are formed by the combination of blastomeres of differing genotype.

In Vitro Fertilization

In-Vitro Fertilization of Rabbit Follicular Oocytes in Tubal Fluid

SHUETU SUZUKI, M.D., and LUIGI MASTROIANNI, Jr., M.D.

SINCE THE FIRST ATTEMPT at in-vitro fertilization in 1878,[24] various approaches to this problem have been reported in the literature. In the majority of earlier studies, epididymal or ejaculated spermatozoa and ova collected from ovarian follicles or fallopian tubes were used. Following discovery of the capacitation phenomenon,[1, 2, 6] results were markedly improved by the use of capacitated spermatozoa. Nevertheless, Austin,[3] in a review of the field up to 1961, concluded that success was most likely attained only by Smith,[25, 26] Moricard,[14] Dauzier et al.,[10] Thibault et al.,[29] Dauzier and Thibault,[11] Chang,[9] and Thibault and Dauzier.[30] More recently, successful in-vitro fertilization has been reported by Bedford and Chang,[4] Yanagimachi and Chang,[32, 33] Suzuki and Mastroianni,[28] and Brackett and Williams.[5] These investigators have employed ova recovered from the fallopian tubes.

The purpose of the present investigation was to assess fertilization of rabbit follicular oocytes under a variety of in-vitro conditions.

MATERIALS AND METHODS

New Zealand White rabbits weighing 3–5 kg. were used. Ovaries were removed and placed in a sterile watch glass containing freshly collected tubal fluid. Large follicles were punctured with a fine needle, and their contents were expressed into a watch glass under a dissecting microscope. Oocytes, surrounded by a thick layer of follicular cells, were easily picked up with a fine pipet. They were transferred promptly to another watch glass containing warm tubal fluid and washed 2 or 3 times. Tubal fluid was harvested from oviducts of adult rabbits, previously ligated at both ends. One drop of uterine fluid containing progressive, motile spermatozoa,

Supported by Grant HD 01810 from the U. S. Public Health Service and by the Ford Foundation.

collected from the uterine cavity by aspiration 12 hr. after mating, was mixed with 2–3 ml. of freshly collected tubal fluid and incubated in a tuberculin syringe at 37° C. for 15 min. before use. Ova were placed in 1–2 drops of tubal fluid in depression slides, and approximately 3 times the volume of sperm suspension was added. After thorough mixing, this suspension was covered with warmed mineral oil and incubated at 37° C. in 5% CO_2 in air. The mineral oil had been mixed with Waymouth's tissue culture medium* in a ratio of 20:1, and the mixture equilibrated with 5% CO_2 in air. After 4 hr., ova were gently washed in a depression slide with tissue culture medium and placed in groups of 5–7 in small Carrel flasks containing 1 ml. of Waymouth's medium, to which 10% rabbit serum had been added. After the flask was gassed with 5% CO_2 in air for 15 min., it was sealed with a rubber stopper and cultured for 8–10 or 18–26 hr. at 37° C. Individual ova were then placed in the center of 4 Vaseline spots on a slide. A coverslip was placed over each ovum and gently compressed until structures within the ovum were clearly visible under the phase-contrast microscope. Ova were photographed, and representative ova were formalin-fixed and stained with acetic lacmoid for further study. Throughout this experiment, aseptic procedures were used and all glassware was sterilized and warmed before and during use.

In 10 series of experiments the conditions were modified as follows:

Series A   Follicular oocytes were collected from rabbits treated intravenously with 100 I.U. human chorionic gonadotropin 8 hr. before. Incubation was carried out in tubal fluid collected from oviducts doubly ligated 4–5 days earlier.

Series B   Oocytes were collected as in Series A, but pretreated with 0.1% hyaluronidase for 10 min. before insemination. Incubation was carried out in tubal fluid collected as in Series A.

Series C   Oocytes were collected as in Series A. The tubal fluid used was collected from oviducts which had been ligated 8 hr. after administration of 200 I.U. of human chorionic gonadotropin.

Series D   Oocytes and tubal fluid were collected as in Series C, but oocytes were treated with 0.1% hyaluronidase for 10 min. before insemination.

Series E   Both oocytes and tubal fluid were collected as in Series C, but prior to insemination oocytes were incubated in vitro for 14–16 hr. in Waymouth's medium containing 10% rabbit serum.

Series F   Oocytes and tubal fluid were collected as in Series A, but prior to insemination oocytes were incubated in the fallopian tubes of the same rabbit in vivo for 1 hr.

---

*Baltimore Biological Laboratories, Baltimore, Md.

Series G   Tubal fluid was collected as in Series A, but the oocytes were recovered from ovarian follicles of rabbits injected with 100 I.U. human chorionic gonadotropin 12 hr. before.

Series H   Oocytes were collected as in Series G, but washing and insemination were carried out in Krebs-Ringer bicarbonate solution with or without 10% rabbit serum.

Series I   Oocytes were collected as in Series G, but ova were washed in Krebs-Ringer bicarbonate solution, and insemination was carried out in Krebs-Ringer bicarbonate solution containing the protein fraction of rabbit tubal fluid (2.0–2.2 mg./ml.). To recover the protein fraction, freshly collected tubal fluid was passed through Sephadex G-25 with NH_4HCO_3 (0.04 M) as a buffer. Once a sample was applied to the column, it was left to equilibrate for 2 hr. Fractions were identified by spectrophotometric scanning at 254 mμ and then lyophilized to dryness.

Series J-E and J-G   Experiments were carried out as in Series E and Series G, but ova were removed from culture 8–10 hr. after insemination.

Ova incubated for 18–24 hr. (Table 1) were classified into 4 groups, essentially according to the criteria suggested by Chang[9] (Table 1): (1) definitely unfertilized—these ova displayed a first polar body in the perivitelline space and a second maturation spindle; (2) degenerating but possibly fertilized—these ova did not display a second maturation spindle, and they contained one or more structures resembling pronuclei; (3) degenerating but probably fertilized—these ova had some spermatozoa in the zona pellucida or in the perivitelline space, and a few showed evidence of impending cleavage but displayed signs of degeneration or fragmentation; (4) normally cleaved and definitely fertilized—these ova were at the two- or more cell stage, and the cells were apparently normal.

TABLE 1. Status of Rabbit Follicular Ova Inseminated in Tubal Fluid (Series A through G), or Artificial Media (H and I) and Cultured for 16–24 Hr.

Series	No. of ova studied	Definitely unfertilized (%)	Possibly fertilized (%)	Probably fertilized (%)	Fertilized; 2 or more cells (%)
A	34	33 (97.1)	0	1 (2.9)	0
B	29	25 (86.2)	4 (13.8)	0	0
C	62	56 (90.3)	2 (3.2)	4 (6.5)	0
D	21	19 (90.5)	0	2 (9.5)	0
E	70	50 (71.4)	6 (8.6)	4 (5.7)	10 (14.3)
F	29	29 (100)	0	0	0
G	74	44 (59.5)	4 (5.4)	5 (6.2)	21 (28.9)
H	28	28 (100)	0	0	0
I	19	19 (100)	0	0	0

TABLE 2. Status of Rabbit Follicular Ova Inseminated in Tubal Fluid and Cultured for 8–10 Hr.

Series	No. of ova studied	Unfertilized; degenerated ova included	Sperm in zona or perivitelline space	Fertilized; 2 pronuclei and 2 polar bodies (%)
J–E	27	20	3	4 (14.5)
J–G	31	18	4	9 (28.7)

Ova incubated for 8–10 hr. following insemination (Table 2) were classified as displaying: (1) no signs of fertilization—degenerated or fragmented ova were included; (2) sperm in the zona pellucida or perivitelline space, 1 or 2 polar bodies in evidence; (3) 2 well-developed pronuclei and 2 polar bodies, interpreted as being definitely fertilized.

RESULTS

A total of 424 ova was used in this study (Tables 1 and 2). In-vitro fertilization of follicular ova was successful when tubal fluid was used, but only when collection of ova was delayed until 12 hr. after gonadotropin treatment (Series G and J-G), or when ova obtained 8 hr. after gonadotropin stimulation were incubated to allow further maturation prior to insemination (Series E and J-E). Ova recovered 12 hr. after gonadotropin stimulation and inseminated in Krebs-Ringer bicarbonate solution were unfertilized (Series H). The protein fraction of tubal fluid failed to influence the fertilization rate (Series I). No fertilization was observed among ova recovered 8 hr. after gonadotropin treatment, with or without pretreatment with hyaluronidase (Series A, B, C, and D), or when such ova were incubated for 1 hr. in the fallopian tubes prior to insemination (Series F). Representative ova are shown in Fig. 1 to 6.

DISCUSSION

In the majority of recent reports on in-vitro fertilization, ovulated ova recovered from the fallopian tubes were used. In work reported before the capacitation phenomenon was discovered, attempts at in-vitro fertilization of follicular ova used ejaculated or epididymal spermatozoa. In the primate, the capacitation phenomenon has not been documented, although cleavage of human ova following exposure to ejaculated semen has been reported by several workers.[13, 23, 24, 34] In the rabbit, several investigators have attempted in-vitro fertilization of follicular ova.[12, 15–21, 23, 31] In each case, however, ejaculated or epididymal spermatozoa were used, and any claim of success should be interpreted with this in mind. In the present

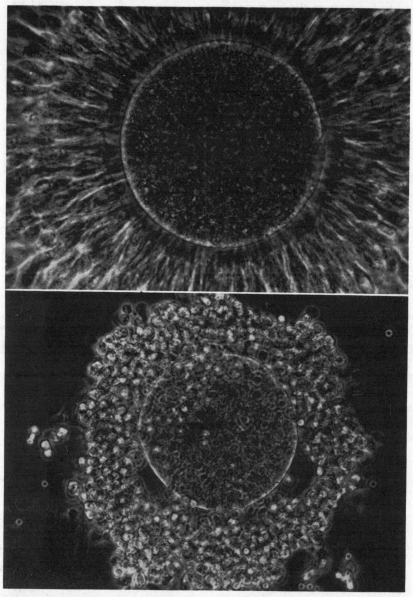

Fig. 1 *(top).* Follicular ovum recovered 12 hr. after gonadotropin treatment (Series G). Note compact layer of granulosa cells. (× 560) **Fig. 2** *(bottom).* Follicular ovum recovered 8 hr. after gonadotropin treatment and cultured for 1 hr. in fallopian tube of same rabbit prior to insemination in vitro (Series F). Superficial layers of granulosa cells are dispersed, leaving compact corona radiata layer which precludes identification of first polar body. (× 560)

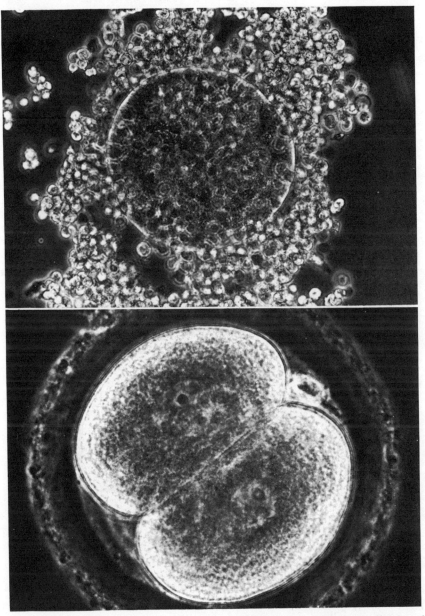

Fig. 3 *(top)*. Follicular ovum recovered 8 hr. after gonadotropin treatment and cultured for 14 hr. in vitro prior to insemination (Series E). (× 560) **Fig. 4** *(bottom)*. Ovum in 2-cell stage. Nuclei are visible in each cell. Inseminated in vitro in tubal fluid and cultured for 20 hr. after insemination (Series G). (× 900)

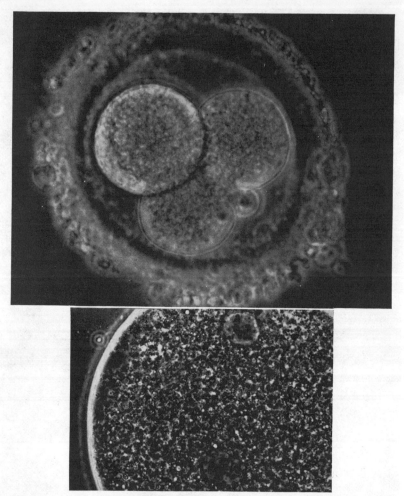

Fig. 5 *(top)*. Ovum in 3-cell stage. Inseminated in vitro in tubal fluid and cultured for 26 hr. after insemination (Series E). (× 560) **Fig. 6** *(bottom)*. Ovum recovered from follicle 8 hr. after gonadotropin treatment, cultured for 14 hr. in vitro prior to insemination, and then incubated for 8 hr. in tubal fluid in vitro with capacitated sperm (Series J-E). Note 2 well-developed pronuclei. (× 1200)

series, in-vitro fertilization of follicular ova was successful. The common denominators were twofold: (1) Tubal fluid was used as a medium, and (2) mature follicular ova recovered from follicles of rabbits treated with gonadotropin 12 hr. before, or ova removed 8 hr. after gonadotropin stimulation and cultured in vitro to allow further maturation prior to insemination, were used. Attempts at in-vitro fertilization in other than whole tubal fluid (Krebs-Ringer bicarbonate solution with and without rabbit serum, or with added protein fraction of rabbit tubal fluid) were unsuccessful, nor was in-vitro fertilization observed when ova from animals which received gonadotropin 8 hr. before were inseminated immediately after recovery. The continued influence of follicular environment, with its known effect on the relationship between the corona cells and zona pellucida,[35, 36] may induce additional ovular changes prerequisite to fertilization. That such changes can proceed at some point in time outside of the follicle is suggested by the observation that ova removed 8 hr. after gonadotropin treatment are fertilizable if cultured in vitro for 14–16 hr.

In earlier experiments, a high success rate was attained when tubal ova were incubated in tubal fluid with capacitated spermatozoa.[27, 28] Tubal fluid was also used in the present study, and it would appear to be a suitable medium for fertilization in vitro. Nevertheless, the success rate with follicular ova is considerably lower than that observed with tubal ova, suggesting that the in-vitro conditions necessary to effect fertilization of follicular ova are more difficult to control. The fertilized follicular ova were not previously exposed to the tubal environment in vivo.

Fertilization of rabbit tubal ova in vitro has been accomplished in various artificial media. Such ova had, of course, had some exposure to the lumen of the fallopian tube. Fertilization of rabbit follicular ova has been reported, but only when they have been placed in the fallopian tubes after they were removed from the follicles.[7, 8] The approach used in this study provides a model for assessing the influence, if any, of the individual components of the tubal environment on the mammalian fertilization process.

SUMMARY

A total of 424 ovarian follicular oocytes of the rabbit was inseminated in vitro with capacitated spermatozoa recovered from the uterine cavity 12 hr. after mating. In-vitro fertilization of follicular ova was accomplished in tubal fluid when collection of ova was delayed until 12 hr. after chorionic gonadotropin stimulation, or when ova obtained 8 hr. after gonadotropin treatment were incubated to allow further maturation prior to insemination. Attempts at in-vitro fertilization in other than tubal fluid were unsuccessful. No fertilization was observed when ova were inseminated immediately after recovery 8 hr. after gonadotropin treatment. The protein fraction of tubal fluid failed to influence the fertilization rate.

REFERENCES

1. AUSTIN, C. R. Observations on the penetration of the sperm into the mammalian egg. *Aust J Sci Res* Ser. B 4:581, 1951.
2. AUSTIN, C. R. The "capacitation" of the mammalian sperm. *Nature 170:*326, 1952.
3. AUSTIN, C. R. Fertilization of mammalian eggs in vitro. *Int Rev Cytol 12:*337, 1961.
4. BEDFORD, J. M., and CHANG, M. C. Fertilization of rabbit ova in vitro. *Nature 193:*898, 1962.
5. BRACKETT, B. G., and WILLIAMS, W. L. In vitro fertilization of rabbit ova. *J Exp Zool 160:*271, 1965.
6. CHANG, M. C. Fertilizing capacity of spermatozoa deposited into the fallopian tubes. *Nature 168:*697, 1951.
7. CHANG, M. C. The maturation of rabbit oocytes in culture and their maturation, activation, fertilization and subsequent development in the fallopian tubes. *J Exp Zool 128:*379, 1955.
8. CHANG, M. C. Fertilization and normal development of follicular oocytes in the rabbit. *Science 121:*867, 1955.
9. CHANG, M. C. Fertilization of rabbit ova in vitro. *Nature 184:*466, 1959.
10. DAUZIER, L., THIBAULT, C., and WINTENBERGER, S. La fécondation in vitro de l'oeuf de la lapine. *C R Acad Sci (Paris) 238:*844, 1954.
11. DAUZIER, L., and THIBAULT, C. Donnes nouvelles sur la fécondation in vitro de l'oeuf de la lapine et de la brebis. *C R Acad Sci (Paris) 248:*2655, 1959.
12. HAYASHI, M., YANG, W. H., and AMANO, E. Fertilization in vitro of rabbit follicular ova. *Asian Med J 7:*757, 1964.
13. MENKIN, M. F., and ROCK, J. In vitro fertilization and cleavage of human ovarian eggs. *Amer J Obstet Gynec 55:*440, 1948.
14. MORICARD, R. Observation of in vitro fertilization in the rabbit. *Nature 173:*1140, 1954.
15. PINCUS, G. Observation on the living eggs of the rabbit. *Proc Roy Soc [Biol] 107:*132, 1930.
16. PINCUS, G. *The Eggs of Mammals.* Macmillan, New York, 1936.
17. PINCUS, G. The comparative behavior of mammalian eggs in vivo and in vitro. IV. The development of fertilized and artificially activated rabbit eggs. *J Exp Zool 82:*85, 1939.
18. PINCUS, G., and ENZMANN, E. V. Can mammalian eggs undergo normal development in vitro? *Proc Nat Acad Sci USA 20:*121, 1934.
19. PINCUS, G., and ENZMANN, E. V. The comparative behavior of mammalian eggs in vivo and in vitro. I. The activation of ovarian eggs. *J Exp Med 62:*665, 1935.
20. PINCUS, G., and ENZMANN, E. V. The comparative behavior of mammalian eggs in vivo and in vitro. II. The activation of tubal eggs of the rabbit. *J Exp Zool 73:* 195, 1936.
21. PINCUS, G., and ENZMANN, E. V. The growth, maturation and atresia of ovarian eggs in the rabbit. *J Morph 61:*351, 1937.
22. ROCK, J., and MENKIN, M. F. In vitro fertilization and cleavage of human ovarian eggs. *Science 100:*105, 1944.
23. SCHENK, S. L. Das Saügethierei künstlich befruchtet ausserhalb des Mutterthieres. *Mitt Embryol Inst K K Univ Wien 1:*107, 1878.
24. SHETTLES, L. B. Observations on human follicular and tubal ova. *Amer J Obstet Gynec 66:*235, 1953.

25. Smith, A. U. Cultivation of rabbit eggs and cumuli for phase-contrast microscopy. *Nature (London) 164:*1136, 1949.
26. Smith, A. U. Fertilization in vitro of the mammalian egg. *Biochem Soc Symp 7:* 3, 1951.
27. Suzuki, S., and Mastroianni, L. In-vitro fertilization of rabbit ova in tubal fluid. *Amer J Obstet Gynec 93:*465, 1965.
28. Suzuki, S. In-vitro cultivation of rabbit ova following in vitro fertilization in tubal fluid. *Cytologia 31:*416, 1966.
29. Thibault, C., Dauzier, L., and Wintenberger, S. Étude cytologique de la fécondation in vitro de l'oeuf de la lapine. *C R Soc Biol (Paris) 148:*789, 1954.
30. Thibault, C., and Dauzier, L. Analyse des conditions de la fécondation "in vitro" de l'œuf de la lapine. *Ann Biol Anim Biochim Biophys 1:*277, 1961.
31. Venge, O. "Experiments on Fertilization of Rabbit Ova in Vitro with Subsequent Transfer to Alien Does." In *Mammalian Germ Cells.* Wolstenholme, G. E. W., Ed. Little, Boston, 1953, p. 243.
32. Yanagimachi, R., and Chang, M. C. Fertilization of hamster eggs in vitro. *Nature (London) 200:*281, 1963.
33. Yanagimachi, R., and Chang, M. C. In-vitro fertilization of golden hamster ova. *J Exp Zool 156:*361, 1964.
34. Yang, W. H. The nature of human follicular ova and fertilization in vitro. *J Jap Obstet Gynec 15:*121, 1963.
35. Zamboni, L., Hongsanand, C., and Mastroianni, L. Influence of tubal secretions on rabbit tubal ova. *Fertil Steril 16:*177, 1965.
36. Zamboni, L., and Mastroianni, L. Electron microscopic studies on rabbit ova I. The follicular oocyte. *J Ultrastruct Res 14:*95, 1966.

Fertilization of Rabbit Ova in a Defined Medium

BENJAMIN G. BRACKETT, D.V.M., Ph.D., and
WILLIAM L. WILLIAMS, Ph.D.

IN PREVIOUS EXPERIMENTS it was found that 73% of the recovered ova were fertilized in vitro following incubation with capacitated spermatozoa when uterine fluid recovered with the spermatozoa was present.[2] In these experiments the gametes were handled under paraffin oil at 39° C. with 96–97 percent relative humidity in a medium containing serum. Experiments reported here were directed toward eliminating the requirements of high relative humidity and the presence of biologic fluids of unknown composition in the fertilization medium.

MATERIALS AND METHODS

All experiments were performed similarly to those which yielded the best results previously,[2] but without high relative humidity in all cases. In these experiments 25, 75, or 100 I.U. of HCG (APL* or Pregnyl†) was injected intravenously into a capacitator and into two ovum donors to induce ovulation. Under paraffin oil, ova were flushed from the oviducts 12½ hr. later into 10-cm.-diameter beaker covers. Manipulations of the gametes were done in a warm room at 37–38° C. Capacitated spermatozoa were recovered in 3.0 ml. of 5% serum solution or in 3.0 ml. of defined medium, according to the experiment. The 5% serum solution was com-

Supported in part by Postdoctoral Fellowship 5 F2 HD-15,861-03 from the National Institute of Child Health and Human Development, Grant FR00340-01, Research Career Program Award 2-K3-GM483, and Research Grant GM 10034 from the Division of General Medical Sciences, U. S. Public Health Service.

The authors gratefully acknowledge the technical assistance of Mrs. Eva Kelly.
*Ayerst Laboratories, New York, N. Y.
†Organon, Inc., West Orange, N. J.

posed of acidic saline with 50 U. of penicillin "G," U.S.P., per milliliter,* 0.25% glucose, and 5% heated rabbit serum. The defined medium† consisted of acidic saline, 0.25% glucose, 0.31% sodium bicarbonate, and 0.30% crystalline bovine serum albumin. The concentration of sodium bicarbonate (37×10^{-3} M) was sufficient to maintain a pH of 7.8 under 5% CO_2.

The sperm suspension was put into the incubation vessel, usually either a sealable-type tissue-culture dish, 45×20 mm. (Bellco Glass, Inc.) or 25-ml.-capacity, 50×14 mm. Carrel flask (Clay Adams). An additional volume of 2.0 ml. of medium was added and a volume of 0.5 ml. was removed for sperm counting, motility, and pH determination. The solution (4.5 ml.) was then covered with oil. After ova were added, enough oil was added to nearly fill all air space. A rubber stopper was tightly lodged in the neck of the Carrel flasks. Incubation was carried out at 37–38° C. After 4½ hr. the ova were transferred to 4.5 ml. of 10% serum solution, i.e., acidic saline with 50 U. of penicillin per milliliter, 0.25% glucose, and 10% heated rabbit serum in tissue-culture dishes or small Petri dishes (60×15 mm.) under oil. Incubation in this medium was continued for 18 hr. At this time ova were examined for evidence of fertilization.

Criteria of fertilization used in this work were normal cleavage and the presence of spermatozoa around the ova; representative ova were examined for nuclei in each blastomere, and the presence of chromatin in each blastomere was ascertained in representative ova by staining with lacmoid.

Experiments in Which Fertilization Medium Contained Serum

Several experiments were done in order to determine (1) if fertilization could be accomplished without a high-relative- humidity atmosphere, and then (2) if the requirement of high relative humidity could be replaced by increased CO_2 tension. The fertilization medium used in these experiments was 5% serum solution. Uterine fluid recovered from a doe with hydrometritis and stored at $-10°$ C. until use (stored uterine fluid) was added in some experiments. Inclusion of this fluid in earlier experiments afforded 32% in vitro fertilization.[2] Bicarbonate was added in some experiments to maintain a constant pH under 5% CO_2. In some experiments 0.9–1.8 ml. of fresh uterine fluid was recovered with the spermatozoa from the capacitator's uterine horns, and the fresh uterine fluid therefore composed 18–36% of the total volume (4.5 ml.) of the fertilization medium.

---

*To make acidic saline (pH 4.8), add the following to distilled water: NaCl, 8.800 gm./L.; KCl, 0.300 gm./L.; CaCl₂, 0.250 gm./L.; NaH₂PO₄, 0.105 gm./L.; MgCl₂, 0.025 gm./L.; and penicillin "G," 50 U./ml.

†The defined, or fertilization, medium (pH 7.8 under 5% CO₂) is prepared just before use as follows: Combine 62.5 mg. glucose, 75.0 mg. crystalline bovine serum albumin, and 77.6 mg. sodium bicarbonate; make up to 25 ml. with acidic saline.

Experiments in Which Fertilization Medium Contained No Serum

Other experiments were done to learn (1) whether the requirement of high relative humidity could be replaced by a lowered O_2 tension, and (2) if the biologic fluids, especially the uterine fluid, which had to be fresh and present in large amounts, could be replaced by chemically defined constituents. The defined medium and the paraffin oil used to cover it were equilibrated with 5% CO_2 in N_2 just before use. The medium (25 ml.) was kept in a small (25 ml.) Erlenmeyer flask, tightly stoppered with a serum bottle cap. Syringes used for sperm recovery and ovum flushing were filled from the Erlenmeyer flask and as a result some air was introduced into the solution. In these experiments tightly stoppered 25-ml.-capacity Carrel flasks were used for the gamete incubation and small Petri dishes were used for culture of the newly fertilized ova.

RESULTS

Ova from 83 New Zealand White does were studied. Of a total of 619 ova predicted by counting ovulation points on the ovaries, 432 were found in these experiments and are accounted for in this report. The over-all recovery of ova predicted was therefore 70%.

Experiments in Which Fertilization Medium Contained Serum

Fertilization Without Added CO_2. These experiments were designed to determine if fertilization could take place without control of the composition of the atmosphere. In two experiments stored uterine fluid was added to the medium. None of 13 ova was fertilized whereas 14 of 16 control ova fertilized in vivo (88%) developed normally. In another experiment the fertilization medium included 9% uterine fluid. This uterine fluid was gained with capacitated spermatozoa in calcium-free Krebs-Ringer phosphate containing 0.25% glucose and 5% heated rabbit serum. The spermatozoa were removed and the solution was stored at $-10°$ C. until use. One of eight ova (13%) was fertilized, but it ceased to develop beyond the two-cell stage. Four of five (80%) control ova developed normally. The fertilization media of these experiments contained $\sim 14 \times 10^4$ spermatozoa per milliliter.

Fertilization Medium Exposed to 5% CO_2 in Air. Three experiments were done to determine if fertilization might be enhanced by exposing the medium directly to a 5%-CO_2-in-air atmosphere. In these experiments the gametes were handled initially at temperatures between 30 and 38° C. The 5% serum solution and paraffin oil were equilibrated with 5% CO_2 in air just before use. Paraffin oil was used in these three experiments only during recovery of ova. Ova were placed in the sperm suspension (2.0–18 × 10⁴ spermatozoa per milliliter) in 10-ml.-capacity unstoppered Carrel flasks and incubated at 38° C. under 5% CO_2 in air. In two of these experiments stored uterine fluid made up 40–50% of the medium of pH 7.8. In these three experiments the ova were not transferred to 10% serum solution but were left with the spermatozoa in the 5% serum solution for the duration of the experiment.

In the first experiment none of 13 experimental ova was fertilized, and none of 10 control ova cleaved. This failure was attributed to a drop of pH from near neutrality to 6.5 during incubation. This situation was corrected in the next two experiments by inclusion of sufficient bicarbonate in the medium to maintain neutrality. However, in the next two experiments results were not greatly improved; only 1 of 25 experimental ova (4%) was fertilized and developed to the four-cell stage, and none of 6 control ova cleaved.

Fertilization under Paraffin Oil Equilibrated with 5% CO_2. Six experiments were performed to determine if a high proportion of ova could be fertilized in media subjected to treatment with 5% CO_2 in air. Various combinations of the solutions composing the fertilization media were equilibrated with 5% CO_2 in air just before use (Table 1). All media were covered by paraffin

TABLE 1. Fertilization under Paraffin Oil Equilibrated with 5% CO_2 in Air

Exp. No.	Variables	In vitro fertilization		In vivo fertilization	
		Ova cleaved/ ova recovered	% normal cleavage	Ova cleaved/ ova recovered	% normal cleavage
9–34	Fresh uterine fluid	5/8	63	8/8	100
9–45	5% CO_2-in-air-equilibrated stored uterine fluid and 5% CO_2-in-air-equilibrated 5% serum solution	1/1	100	0/7	0
9–54	Fresh uterine fluid and 5% CO_2-in-air-equilibrated 5% serum solution	0/12	0	8/8	100
9–37	Fresh uterine fluid and stored uterine fluid	0/6	0	5/6	84
9–48	Fresh uterine fluid and 5% CO_2-in-air-equilibrated stored uterine fluid and 5% CO_2-in-air-equilibrated 5% serum solution	1/8	13	8/8	100
9–51		0/9	0	4/4	100
	TOTALS AND AVERAGES	7/44	16	33/41	81

oil through which 5% CO_2 in air was bubbled just before use. The results are indicated in Table 1. Fertilization media in these experiments contained 2.2–68 $\times$ 10^4 spermatozoa per milliliter.

In Experiment 9–45 (Table 1) the pH of the control medium was 6.3 during the initial incubation, a level that was probably too acid to support development of ova. In other controls stored uterine fluid was included in the medium to stabilize the pH. Under similar conditions none of 32 ova cleaved as a result of incubation without spermatozoa. This control experiment ruled out any consideration of parthenogenetic development and degenerative fragmentation.

In one experiment the paraffin oil was equilibrated with 5% CO_2 in N_2. The fertilization medium contained 36% fresh uterine fluid and 19$\times$ 10^4 spermatozoa per milliliter. Eleven of 14 ova (79%) were fertilized in vitro. Five of the six control ova developed normally. In contrast to Experiment No. 9–34 (Table 1), in which 4 of the 5 in-vitro fertilized ova cleaved only once, all ova fertilized in this experiment developed normally. This finding suggested that a reduction of O_2 tension might favor fertilization and early development of ova in vitro.

Experiments in Which Fertilization Medium Contained No Serum

Fertilization with Fresh Uterine Fluid Comprising 18–44% of Medium. In four experiments a measurable volume (0.8–2.0 ml.) of uterine fluid was recovered with the capacitated spermatozoa (Table 2). In these experiments the uterine fluid was the only constituent of the fertilization medium which was not chemically defined. It comprised 18–44% of the volume of the fertilization medium. Sperm concentrations in these experiments ranged from 32 to 75 $\times$ 10^4 spermatozoa per milliliter. Results of these experiments are shown in Table 2. A consistently high rate of fertilization was

TABLE 2. Fertilization with Fresh Uterine Fluid in the Medium

Exp. No.	In vitro fertilization		In vivo fertilization	
	Ova cleaved/ ova recovered	% normal cleavage	Ova cleaved/ ova recovered	% normal cleavage
9–72	8/12	67	5/5	100
12–34	10/12	83	3/3	100
12–36	5/6	83	2/2	100
12–38	7/15*	47*	3/3	100
TOTALS AND AVERAGES	30/45	67	13/13	100

*Ovum donors were lactating; Waymouth's medium was used for ovum culture.

observed. Representative in-vitro fertilized ova from Experiment No. 12–34 were photographed (Fig. 1–3). Spermatozoa were generally quite motile at the end of an experiment, and the sperm cell pictured in Fig. 2 was still active 8 hr. after the end of the experiment ($\sim$ 44 hr. after ejaculation),

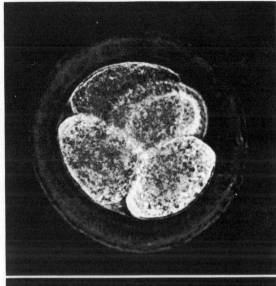

Fig. 1. Representative in-vitro fertilized ovum from Experiment No. 12–34. (Phase contrast, $\times$ 560)

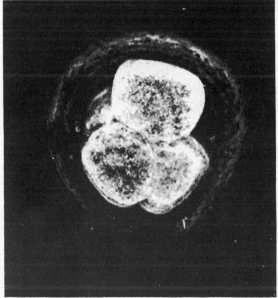

Fig. 2. In-vitro fertilized ovum with adhering sperm cell from Experiment No. 12–34. (Phase contrast, $\times$ 560)

when it was photographed. Ova in these cultures often assumed a flattened appearance enabling one to see all four blastomeres (Fig. 3).

Seven of the in-vitro fertilized ova ceased to develop beyond the two-cell stage and only one of the control ova stopped at this stage. Five of the two-cell-stage in-vitro fertilized ova were from Experiment No. 12–38, in which Waymouth's medium (Difco) under a 5% CO_2 in air atmosphere

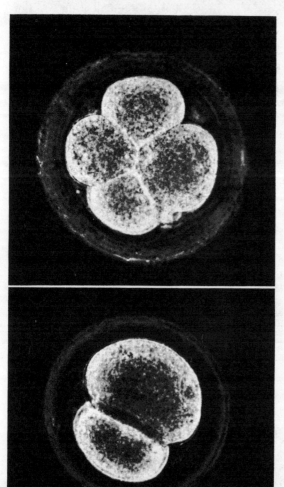

Fig. 3. In-vitro fertilized ovum that has become flattened in culture. (Phase contrast, × 560)

Fig. 4. In-vitro fertilized ovum from Experiment No. 12–41 infected with bacteria inside the perivitelline space. (Phase contrast, × 560)

was substituted for the usual 10% serum solution culture medium. Also, the ovum donors of this experiment were lactating.

Fertilization in Defined Medium. Six experiments were done in which no measurable volume of uterine fluid was recovered with spermatozoa taken from the uterus of the capacitator. In these experiments $6.0–46 \times 10^4$ spermatozoa were present in each milliliter of the fertilization medium.

In one of these experiments (No. 12–41) the initial incubation was done in an anaerobic bacterial chamber which contained 8% O_2, 5% CO_2, and the balance N_2. The gametes were incubated in small Petri dishes to permit equilibration with the atmosphere. Results of this experiment (Table 3) indicate that 8% O_2 tension is compatible with fertilization in vitro. Four of the in-vitro fertilized ova and one of the control ova in these experiments (Table 3) did not develop beyond the two-cell stage. Two of the in-vitro fertilized ova which cleaved only once were from Experiment No. 12–41. Motile bacteria were found in the perivitelline space of these ova (Fig. 4) and were probably the cause of their death. The proportion of ova fertilized under these conditions is comparable to that of previous experiments in which uterine fluid was a major component of the fertilization medium. A four-cell in-vitro fertilized ovum from Experiment No. 12–27 was depressed under a cover slip to make the four nuclei visible under phase-contrast microscopy (Fig. 5). In a control experiment in which no spermatozoa were present in the fertilization medium, none of 13 ova cleaved or fragmented.

Even though a measurable volume of uterine fluid was not present in the fertilization medium of these experiments, unidentified soluble substances derived from tubal and uterine washings may still have been present. In two experiments the spermatozoa were washed following their recovery.

TABLE 3. Fertilization in a Defined Medium

Exp. No.	In vitro fertilization		In vivo fertilization	
	Ova cleaved/ ova recovered	% normal cleavage	Ova cleaved/ ova recovered	% normal cleavage
9–70	12/16	75	2/2	100
12–21	5/8	63	9/10	90
12–23	4/5	80	2/5*	40*
12–27	4/8	50	6/6	100
12–32	4/6	67	9/9	100
12–41	6/11	55	3/3	100
TOTALS AND AVERAGES	35/54	65	31/35	89

*Initial incubation under 5% CO_2 in air.

The washing procedure consisted of centrifuging the recovered sperm suspension at 200 g for 5 min. The supernatant fluid was discarded and the spermatozoa were resuspended in a fresh volume of defined medium. The ova were added to this fertilization medium. The sperm concentration

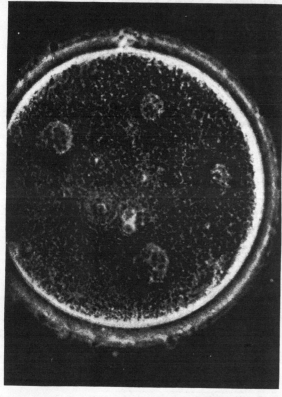

Fig. 5. In-vitro fertilized ovum from Experiment No. 12–27 depressed under cover slip, making nuclei visible. (Phase contrast, × 716)

was 14 or 20 × 10⁴ spermatozoa per milliliter. An additional control was included in one of these experiments in which sperm suspensions from two capacitators were pooled, then divided into two samples. One of these samples was washed and the other was used as an unwashed control. Ova in cumulus clots from three donors were transferred to each of the two sperm suspensions so that ova from each donor were present in each fertilization medium.

Results of these preliminary experiments indicated that the procedure used may lower the proportion of ova fertilized. Four of 20 ova were fertilized in vitro, and all failed to develop beyond the two-cell stage. In the unwashed sperm control 1 of 4 ova (25%) developed to the two-cell stage. Fourteen of the capacitators' 15 ova were fertilized, with 3 of these failing to proceed beyond the two-cell stage.

DISCUSSION

Five per cent CO_2 in air did not enhance fertilization in vitro in the experiments reported here. Suzuki and Mastroianni achieved their highest degree of success in the fertilization of rabbit ova in vitro when the gametes were held in a small volume of tubal fluid under paraffin oil equilibrated with 5% CO_2 in air. These findings are not necessarily in conflict because the media, fluid volumes, and technics were different in the two cases.

In view of the experimental results obtained here, it seems that a high oxygen tension is detrimental to the fertilization process. An oxygen tension of 8%, which is the concentration of O_2 found in the rabbit oviduct,[5] was found to be compatible with fertilization in vitro. Results suggest that lowered O_2 tension also favors the development of early cleavage stages. The 5% CO_2 in N_2-equilibrated medium and paraffin oil may, by reducing O_2 tension, allow the gametes to withstand the small temperature variations which were guarded against in previous work by high relative humidity.

With the elimination of the requirement for high relative humidity, the way was clear for replacing the requirements of serum and the large amount of uterine fluid of the in vitro fertilization medium with chemically defined constituents. It has long been known that ova deteriorate less rapidly in vitro when suspended in media containing substances of high molecular weight.[1] This may be the effect of serum. The serum proteins were replaceable by a comparable amount of crystalline bovine serum albumin. In previous in-vitro fertilization experiments the best results were obtained when 20–40% fresh uterine fluid was present, and the pH of the medium was elevated to values higher than 7.5, presumably because of its bicarbonate content. Therefore, bicarbonate was substituted for the requirement of this large volume of fresh uterine fluid in an amount adequate to maintain a pH of 7.8 under a 5% CO_2 atmosphere. Optimal conditions for in-vitro fertilization previously described were duplicated by conditions which make the study of in-vitro fertilization more precise and more convenient.

The use of solutions of known chemical composition in in-vitro-fertilization experiments has been attempted earlier. Chang achieved fertilization of 21% of the ova which he incubated with uterine spermatozoa in Krebs-Ringer bicarbonate solution. Thibault and Dauzier used Locke's solution in their experiments, which resulted in 66% of the ova having either a swell-mg sperm head and midpiece and a second polar body or male and female pronuclei. The conditions found in the present investigation make possible the study of effects of added chemicals on the fertilization process and early cleavage stages in vitro. The next most critical experiment, however, is yet to be done. The spermatozoa and ova must be repeatedly washed to eliminate soluble unidentified substances present in the tubal and uterine washings. The gametes should then be combined in a medium of chemically pure ingredients under proper physical conditions. These experiments are now in progress in our laboratories.

In initial experiments washing of the spermatozoa, following their recovery from the uterus, lowered the proportion of ova fertilized and retarded the development of those which were fertilized. Perhaps the anti-fertilizin-like substance proposed by Thibault and Dauzier was washed from the spermatozoa, resulting in delayed penetration of the ova. This system for in-vitro fertilization may be helpful in elucidating the mechanism of sperm capacitation and sperm penetration of mammalian ova.

REFERENCES

1. AUSTIN, C. R. *The Mammalian Egg.* Blackwell, Oxford, 1963, p. 183.
2. BRACKETT, B. G., and WILLIAMS, W. L. *In vitro* fertilization of rabbit ova. *J Exper Zool 160:*271, 1965.
3. CHANG, M. C. Fertilization of rabbit ova *in vitro. Nature 184:*466, 1959.
4. HAMMOND, J. Recovery and culture cf tubal mouse ova. *Nature 163:*28, 1949.
5. MASTROIANNI, L., and JONES, R. Oxygen tension within the rabbit fallopian tube. *J Reprod Fertil 9:*99, 1965.
6. SUZUKI, S., and MASTROIANNI, L. *In vitro* fertilization of rabbit ova in tubal fluid. *Amer J Obstet Gynec 93:*465, 1965.
7. THIBAULT, C., and DAUZIER, L. Analyse des conditions de la fecondation *in vitro* de l'oeuf de la lapine. *Ann Biol Anim Biochim Biophys 1:*277, 1961.

Effects of Washing the Gametes on Fertilization In Vitro

BENJAMIN G. BRACKETT, D.V.M., PH.D.

PREVIOUS INVESTIGATIONS have made possible the fertilization of a high proportion of rabbit ova following in-vitro incubation with capacitated spermatozoa.[2, 4, 5, 8–12, 14, 15, 17, 19–23] Recent work has been concerned primarily with defining the in-vitro conditions necessary for the fertilization of rabbit ova to occur.[4, 5, 21] The present in-vitro fertilization experiments were designed to study effects of washing the gametes free of female reproductive tract secretions prior to their incubation together in a defined medium.

MATERIALS AND METHODS

These experiments were performed in the fashion of those reported previously.[4, 5] Mature New Zealand White does were caged individually for at least 19 days before use to eliminate the chances of pseudopregnancy. Experiments were initiated by mating a doe (capacitator) with 2–5 fertile males. Then, the capacitator was usually given an injection of 50 or 75 I.U. HCG (A.P.L.* or Pregnyl†) along with 2 other does (ovum donors). In three experiments, ovum donors were superovulated by the procedure used by Brinster,[7] except with a 76-hr. interval between priming and ovula-

Supported by Grant FR 00340-01 from the National Institutes of Health, U. S. Public Health Service and by the Ford Foundation.

The author gratefully acknowledges the technical assistance of Miss S. Arenschield, Mr. and Mrs. N. G. Cole, Jr., Mr. and Mrs. J. Enck, Mrs. E. M. Kelly, and Mr. A. London; and, Mr. J. Butler for care of the animals. The author also acknowledges the assistance of Dr. A. David, in collecting oviduct fluid, Dr. G. L. Flickinger for statistical analyses, and Dr. H. M. Seitz, Jr., in the ovum transfers.
*Ayerst Laboratories, New York, N. Y.
†Orgunon Inc., West Orange, N. J.

tion-inducing injections. Twelve to 13½ hr. later, the does were killed, and the gametes were recovered. Ova were flushed from oviducts under paraffin oil.

Ova from one oviduct of each donor were placed in one tissue culture dish, and ova from the other oviduct were ultimately placed in the other dish (Fig. 1). Capacitated spermatozoa were recovered in 3 or 4 ml. of medium. The sperm suspension was divided, and approximately one-half of the sperm cells were used for incubation with each group of ova. This distribution of gametes from the same animals allowed comparison of results of 2 different treatments in each experiment (Fig. 1). Leukocyte and sperm counts were made directly from fertilization mediums at the beginning of each experiment with a hemocytometer.

The medium used was the defined medium described previously (345 milliosmolar)[5] or the defined medium with the osmolarity adjusted to 280 mosm. by the removal of NaCl to make it more nearly isotonic. A volume of 4 ml. was used for all incubations. The fertilization medium and oil used to cover it were equilibrated with 5% CO_2 in N_2 before use.

The time required for handling the gametes was less than 30 min., and the surrounding air temperature was near 37° C. In most of these experiments, the gametes were incubated initially at 38° C. under air. However, in the best experiments here, as in the best experiments reported

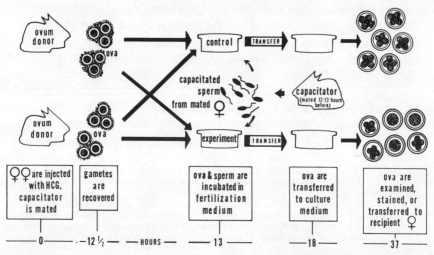

Fig. 1. Schematic diagram of experimental plan for in-vitro fertilization used in these experiments.

32

previously[5] (although not mentioned previously), the gametes were initially incubated under a moist atmosphere of 5% CO_2 in air.

Around 5 hr. after putting ova with spermatozoa, the ova were transferred from the fertilization medium to 10% serum solution previously described (287 milliosmolar),[5] or 10% serum solution with a reduced NaCl content (221 milliosmolar) and cultured an additional 18–20 hr. at 38° C. under 1 atm. The 10% serum solution and paraffin oil used to cover it were in equilibrium with air.

Sealable type, 12- $\times$ 30-mm. size, tissue culture dishes* were used for all incubations. All glassware, syringes, paraffin oil, and mediums were sterile before use.

In some experiments, spermatozoa were washed by centrifugation at 395 $\times$ g for 8 min. Supernatant solutions were discarded, used to resuspend the sperm cells, or saved for use in another experiment. The sperm cells were resuspended by turbulence which was induced by repeated aspiration and expulsion of the suspending fluid with a syringe. In certain experiments, ova were washed by transferring the cumulus clots containing them through 3 different 1-ml. aliquots of the medium under paraffin oil.

Oviduct fluid was used in several experiments. It was collected 4 days after microsurgical ligation of the ampullary region.[13] Osmolarity of the oviduct fluid used, of rabbit serum, and the medium used was determined using an osmette precision osmometer.† Oxygen content of the medium used was determined by a Clark oxygen electrode.‡

In each experiment, ova from the capacitator were recovered and incubated in the same manner as those from the ovum donors. Normal cleavage of these in-vivo fertilized ova indicated that the spermatozoa were capacitated and that the culture conditions were adequate for development of very recently fertilized ova.

Only symmetrically cleaved ova were considered to have been fertilized. Representative ova were stained with lacmoid to verify the presence of chromatin in each blastomere. Proportions of ova fertilized in each experimental series were compared and analyzed statistically by chi-square with Yates correction.

In-vitro fertilized ova from two experiments were surgically transferred to recipient does that were injected with HCG so that they would be in a synchronous hormonal state. Recipients were opened surgically 9 or 10 days following transfer to see whether implantation had taken place. One recipient was retained and allowed to deliver young.

---

*Bellco Glass, Inc., Vineland, N. J.
†Precision Systems, Framingham, Mass.
‡Yellow Springs Instrument Co., Yellow Springs, Ohio.

RESULTS

A total of 945 ova from 146 rabbits were studied. This represents 70% of the 1352 ova shed by these does as estimated by counting ovulation points. Sperm concentrations in these experiments ranged from 6000 to 1,260,-000/ml. of fertilization medium, and sperm motility ranged from 15 to 90%. Leukocytes were invariably carried into the fertilization medium with uterine spermatozoa. Leukocyte concentrations ranged from 26,000 to 7,440,000/ml. and the ratios of leukocytes to sperm cells ranged from 1:1 to 14:1. No correlations could be made between the number of sperm cells or leukocytes to spermatozoa ratios and proportions of ova fertilized in vitro.

Effect of Washing Both Ova and Spermatozoa

These experiments were done to learn whether the removal of soluble substances associated with tubal ova and/or uterine spermatozoa might change the proportion of ova that could be fertilized in vitro. The results are shown in Table 1. Washing both ova and spermatozoa caused a statistically significant ($p < 0.05$) reduction in the proportion of ova that could be fertilized in vitro when both gametes were unwashed. One ovum which was fertilized in vitro in Experiment 12-91 cleaved only once. All the other fertilized ova in Table 1 cleaved to the 4-cell stage by the time of examination.

In Experiment 12-96, three intermediate stage tapeworm larvae (*Cysticercus pisiformis*) were recovered from the oviducts along with ova from the capacitator. The six in-vitro fertilized ova of this experiment were surgically transferred to the right oviduct of a recipient doe that had been

TABLE 1. Effect of Washing Both Ova and Spermatozoa

	In-vitro fertilization		In-vivo fertilization (capacitators' ova)
Exp. No.	Unwashed ova + unwashed spermatozoa	Washed ova + washed spermatozoa	
12-89	3/8*	1/2	9/10
12-91	2/7	0/5	5/5
12-96	5/7	1/6	1/2
12-98	1/3	1/5	2/2
15-118	5/28	0/14	6/7
16-8	3/14	1/11	1/2
Totals	19/67	4/43	24/28
% ova fertil.	28.4	9.3	85.7

* Numerator is the number of ova that cleaved normally; denominator is the number of ova recovered.

given an injection of 75 I.U. HCG 25 hr. earlier. These ova were cultured to the eight-cell stage before transfer. Seven two-cell in-vivo fertilized ova were recovered from a doe that had been mated and given an injection of 75 I.U. HCG 25 hr. earlier. These in-vivo fertilized ova were transferred to the recipient's left oviduct. Five of the in-vitro fertilized ova implanted, but two of the implanted embryos were smaller than normal when examined 10 days after transfer. Two of the in-vivo fertilized ova implanted, but were smaller than normal, indicating resorption at the time of examination. Twenty-eight days after the transfer, the recipient delivered three normal young. She ate two of them soon afterward, but one survived to get his picture taken (Fig. 2).

In Experiments 15-118 and 16-8, the gametes were held under a moist 5% CO_2 in air atmosphere for the first incubation, then cultured overnight under an air atmosphere. The osmolarity of the fertilization medium in these experiments was adjusted to 280 mosm. by decreasing the NaCl content of the salt solution (acidic saline) used. The same salt solution was inadvertently used in preparing the 10% serum solution for ovum culture; therefore, ova which were fertilized in the more nearly isotonic medium (in these and other experiments described below) were cultured in 10% serum solution which was hypotonic, around 221 mosm. In these cultures, fragmented ova were frequently seen. Many of the symmetrically cleaved fertilized ova seemed to be undergoing slight degenerative changes follow-

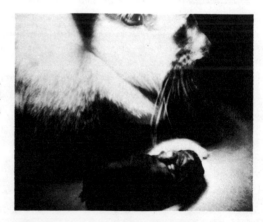

Fig. 2. Normal young developed from ovum fertilized in vitro by spermatozoon from a black buck.

ing culture in media of this osmolarity. In Experiment 16-8, ova which were considered nonfertilized had pronuclei.

Experiments 15-118 and 16-8 also differed from other experiments in this series in the amount of HCG used. Ovum donors of 15-118 were superovulated, and the capacitator was not given any injections. Ovum donors of 16-8 were given 50 I.U. HCG and the capacitator was not injected. In all other experiments of this series, ovum donors and capacitators each were given 75 I.U. HCG.

Effect of Washing Ova Only

Several experiments were done to see if the decrease in the proportion of ova fertilized in vitro, found in the above experiments, was due to washing the ova. Washing the ova enhanced the proportion of ova fertilized in vitro (Table 2). The difference between proportions of washed ova and unwashed ova that were fertilized in these experiments, however, was not statistically significant ($p > 0.05$).

Six of the unwashed ova and 15 of the washed ova that were fertilized failed to develop beyond the two-cell stage. Three of the capacitators' fertilized ova cleaved only once.

In Experiment 12-113, the three in-vitro fertilized ova that were not washed originally were transferred to the left oviduct, and four of the in-vitro fertilized ova that were washed originally were transferred to the right oviduct of a recipient doe. The doe was given an injection of 75 I.U. HCG 22 hr. previously. Nine days later, the recipient was killed, and two normal implants were observed in the right uterine horn.

In Experiments 15-47, 15-55, and 15-57, the capacitators were not given

TABLE 2. Effect of Washing Ova Only

	In-vitro fertilization		In-vivo fertilization (capacitators' ova)
Exp. No.	Unwashed ova + unwashed spermatozoa	Washed ova + unwashed spermatozoa	
12-113	3/7*	5/7	3/7
15-10	1/6	0/3	2/2
15-13	1/3	2/10	5/6
15-27	2/3	0/1	2/2
15-32	1/7	0/5	10/11
15-37	0/7	5/10	4/6
15-43	0/9	1/7	4/4
15-47	6/10	8/10	6/7
15-55	2/4	1/7	—
15-57	0/3	3/6	7/7
Totals	16/59	25/66	43/52
% ova fertil.	27.1	37.8	82.7

* Numerator is the number of ova that cleaved normally; denominator is the number of ova recovered.

36

injections of HCG, but the donors were given 75 I.U. In all other experiments of this group, ovum donors and capacitators were given 75 I.U. HCG.

Effect of Washing Spermatozoa Only

These experiments were done to see if washing the spermatozoa would cause a smaller proportion of ova to be fertilized in vitro than that observed when neither gametes were washed. Results of these experiments (Table 3) indicate that washing the spermatozoa free of uterine secretions caused a statistically significant ($p < 0.05$) decrease in the proportion of ova that could be fertilized in vitro.

Seven of the ova fertilized by unwashed spermatozoa, and five of the ova fertilized by washed spermatozoa developed only to the two-cell stage. Only one of the capacitators' ova stopped at the two-cell stage.

In Experiment 15-115 (I and II) the gametes were incubated initially under a moist 5% CO_2 in air atmosphere and the osmolarity of the fertilization medium was adjusted to 280. In this experiment, all rabbits were given injections of 50 I.U. HCG. In other experiments of this series, the capacitators were not given any HCG.

Effect of Centrifugation of the Spermatozoa

Since washing the spermatozoa reduced the proportion of ova fertilized in vitro, it was of interest to see whether the centrifugation of the sperm cells was responsible for this effect. In these experiments (Table 4), the

TABLE 3. Effect of Washing Spermatozoa Only

| | In-vitro fertilization | | |
Exp. No.	Unwashed ova + unwashed spermatozoa	Unwashed ova + washed spermatozoa	In-vivo fertilization (capacitators' ova)
15-62	5/8*	3/9	4/4
15-64	2/3	0/4	6/6
15-79	2/4	1/2	3/3
15-83-I	3/6	1/9	3/5
15-90	1/1	0/2	6/8
15-95	1/4	1/9	1/2
15-115-I	0/5	1/9	6/7
15-115-II	6/6	7/7	4/4
TOTALS	20/37	14/51	33/39
% ova fertil.	54.0	27.4	84.6

* Numerator is the number of ova that cleaved normally; denominator is the number of ova recovered.

TABLE 4. Effect of Centrifugation of the Spermatozoa

	In-vitro fertilization		In-vivo fertilization (capacitators' ova)
Exp. No.	Unwashed ova + unwashed spermatozoa	Unwashed ova + centrif. spermatozoa	
15-67	1/5*	0/10	—
15-75	3/6	5/9	12/12
15-83-II	4/10	0/9	13/13
15-104-I	3/6	2/6	1/1
15-104-II	4/6	1/6	3/4
15-110-I	9/9	14/18	9/11
15-110-II	10/13	6/8	8/8
Totals	34/55	28/66	46/49
% ova fertil.	61.8	42.4	93.9

* Numerator is the number of ova that cleaved normally; denominator is the number of ova recovered.

proportion of ova fertilized by centrifuged spermatozoa that were resuspended in the washings was compared with the proportion of ova fertilized by unwashed spermatozoa. The proportion of ova fertilized by the centrifuged spermatozoa was not significantly different from the proportion of ova fertilized by unwashed spermatozoa ($p > 0.05$).

In these experiments, four of the unwashed ova fertilized by unwashed spermatozoa, and six of the unwashed ova fertilized by centrifuged spermatozoa developed only to the two-cell stage. Three of the capacitators' ova cleaved only once.

In Experiments 15-67, 15-75, and 15-83-II, the capacitators were not given injections of HCG; the ovum donors were given 75 I.U. HCG. In Experiments 15-104-II and 15-110-I, the gametes were initially incubated under 5% CO_2 in air in the defined medium with the osmolarity adjusted to 280 mosm. In Experiment 15-104-I, the 5% CO_2 in air atmosphere was used initially, but the osmolarity of the fertillization and culture medium was the same as in former experiments.

Experiments 15-104-I and II were done at the same time, but with different rabbits and mediums of differing osmolarities. Ova in Experiment 15-104-I, fertilized and cultured in the usual way, developed to the four-cell stage by the time of examination 26 hr. after putting ova with spermatozoa. Ova in Experiment 15-104-II, fertilized in more nearly isotonic solution and cultured in the hypotonic 10% serum solution, developed to the eight-cell stage by the time of examination, 26 hr. after putting ova with spermatozoa.

Comparison of Results When Only Spermatozoa Were Washed with Those When Both Gametes Were Washed

If the decrease in fertilization of ova observed after washing both gametes was due entirely to an effect on the sperm cells, the proportion of ova fertilized by washed spermatozoa should be the same as that resulting from incubation of washed ova with washed spermatozoa. Data in Table 5 show that this was the case ($p > 0.95$).

Eight of the unwashed ova, and two of the washed ova cleaved only once following fertilization. One of the capacitators' ova cleaved only once.

In Experiments 12-105 (I and II), 12-107, and 12-109, the paraffin oil used initially was not equilibrated with 5% CO_2 in N_2. In Experiments 16-17 and 16-22-I, the gametes were incubated initially under 5% CO_2 in air in 280 milliosmolar fertilization medium and cultured in 221 milliosmolar 10% serum solution under air. Ovum donors of Experiment 16-17 were superovulated.

Effect of Adding Sperm Washings to Washed Spermatozoa

From the preceding experiments, it was apparent that something beneficial to fertilization was being removed from the spermatozoa by washing them. Supernatant solutions were saved after washing spermatozoa in several experiments. These sperm washings were used to resuspend washed spermatozoa in these experiments. The proportion of ova fertilized by washed spermatozoa with sperm washings added might be expected to be greater than the proportion of ova fertilized by washed spermatozoa alone.

TABLE 5. Results When Only Spermatozoa Were Washed and When Both Gametes Were Washed

	In-vitro fertilization		
Exp. No.	Unwashed ova + washed spermatozoa	Washed ova + washed spermatozoa	In-vivo fertilization (capacitators' ova)
12-105-I	0/3*	3/8	4/5
12-105-II	6/9	6/9	4/5
12-107	7/10	1/3	1/1
12-109	0/7	1/7	—
16-17	3/8	1/5	6/8
16-22-I	4/8	8/10	6/6
TOTALS	20/45	20/42	21/25
% ova fertil.	44.4	47.6	84.0

* Numerator is the number of ova that cleaved normally; denominator is the number of ova recovered.

TABLE 6. Effect of Adding Sperm Washings to Washed Spermatozoa

TABLE 6. Effect of Adding Sperm Washings to Washed Spermatozoa

	In-vitro fertilization		
Exp. No.	Washed ova + washed spermatozoa	Washed ova + washed spermatozoa + sperm washings	In-vivo fertilization (capacitators' ova)
16-10	12/17*	1/9	5/5
16-19	0/10	5/10	6/6
16-22-II	3/5	6/11	0/1
Totals	15/32	12/30	11/12
% ova fertil.	46.9	40.0	91.7

* Numerator is the number of ova that cleaved normally; denominator is the number of ova recovered.

Results in Table 6 indicate that the addition of sperm washings to washed spermatozoa did not increase the proportion of ova that could be fertilized over that obtained with washed spermatozoa alone.

Two of the washed ova fertilized by washed spermatozoa and three of the washed ova fertilized by washed spermatozoa with sperm washings added cleaved only once. All control ova cleaved to the four-cell stage by the time of examination. The osmolarity of the fertilization medium used in these experiments was adjusted to 280 mosm. The initial incubation of gametes was under 5% CO_2 in air.

In Experiment 16-10, one superovulated ovum donor was used. The sperm washings in this experiment were stored at $-15°$ C. following collection in Experiment 15-115-II (Table 3) 2 weeks earlier. The volume of washings was only 2.0 ml.; therefore, an additional 2.0 ml. of fertilization medium had to be added to the washed sperm cells to resuspend them to the 4.0 ml. volume used for incubation with ova (see Fig. 3 and 4).

In Experiment 16-19, the sperm washings were refrigerated at 5° C. after collection, which was 2 weeks earlier in Experiment 15-83-I (Table 3). The volume of washings was only 1.5 ml.; therefore an additional 2.5 ml. of fertilization medium had to be added for the desired incubation volume.

In Experiment 16-22-II, the sperm washings were used within 1 hr. after collection in Experiment 16-22-I (Table 5). A measurable volume of fresh uterine fluid (1.0 ml.) was gained with the spermatozoa in Experiment 16-22-I, therefore, uterine secretions definitely contributed to the composition of these washings. These washings were kept warm in a tightly closed syringe until use. The volume of sperm washings in this case was 5.0 ml., so no additional volume of fertilization medium was required.

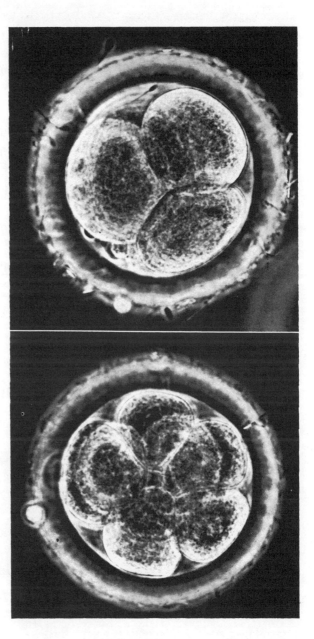

Fig. 3. Four-cell in-vitro fertilized ovum (Experiment 16-10, Table 6) fertilized in vitro in 280 milliosmolar-defined medium and cultured in 221 milliosmolar 10% serum solution.

Fig. 4. Eight-cell in-vitro fertilized ovum (Experiment 16-10, Table 6) fertilized in vitro in 280 milliosmolar-defined medium and cultured in 221 milliosmolar 10% serum solution.

Effect of Adding Ampullary Oviduct Fluid to Washed Spermatozoa

Three experiments were done to see if the addition of ampullary oviduct fluid could enhance the proportion of ova fertilized by washed spermatozoa. The addition of 25% ampullary oviduct fluid to the fertilization medium did not increase the proportion of washed ova that could be fertilized by washed spermatozoa (Table 7).

Two of the ova fertilized in the absence of oviduct fluid, and one of the ova fertilized with oviduct fluid present cleaved only once. One of the capacitators' ova failed to develop beyond this stage.

Each doe in Experiment 12-101 was given an injection of 75 I.U. HCG, whereas a 50-I.U. dose was used for each doe in the other experiments of this group.

Control Ovum Cultures and Observations on Osmolarity

Several experiments were done in which recently ovulated ova were manipulated and incubated as in the above experiments except in the absence of spermatozoa. None of the 101 ova from 15 rabbits cleaved during culture in 10% serum solution (287 milliosmolar) following a 5 hr. incubation in the defined medium (345 milliosmolar). In these experiments, ova were washed or unwashed, incubated with defined medium alone or with uterine washings (in cases where no spermatozoa were recovered), or with oviduct fluid.

Degenerative fragmentation of ova cultured in 10% serum solution with an osmolarity of 221 mosm. was not uncommon. Such fragmented ova were differentiated from symmetrically cleaved fertilized ova by microscopic examination. In contrast to fragmented ova, fertilized ova generally had

TABLE 7. Effect of Adding Ampullary Oviduct Fluid to Washed Spermatozoa

	In-vitro fertilization		
Exp. No.	Washed ova + washed spermatozoa	Washed ova + washed spermatozoa + oviduct fluid	In-vivo fertilization (capacitators' ova)
12-72	3/6*	1/4	0/1
12-75	2/5	2/4	3/6
12-101	6/7	3/3	3/4
Totals	11/18	6/11	6/10
% ova fertil.	61.1	54.6	60.0

* Numerator is the number of ova that cleaved normally; denominator is the number of ova recovered.

spermatozoa present on the zona pellucida or in the perivitelline space (Fig. 3 and 4). Also, lacmoid staining made chromatin apparent in each blastomere of fertilized ova.

Osmolarity of rabbit serum was found to be 279 mosm. and that of oviduct fluid from ligated oviducts was 272 mosm.

Observations on Oxygen Tension

The initial equilibration of media with 5% CO_2 in N_2 served to reduce the O_2 tension of the defined mediums in which fertilization took place. The average O_2 content of 5 of the 345 milliosmolar-defined mediums was 276 μl. O_2/ml. and the range was 2.54–2.91 μl. O_2/ml. These measurements were made on the solutions remaining after beginning the experiments.

In two experiments, 15-110-I and 15-118, in which the 280 milliosmolar-defined medium was used, the O_2 contents of the fertilization medium were determined at the beginning and end of the incubation. Similar values were obtained for the two experiments. For Experiment 15-110-I (Table 4), the initial O_2 content was 2.49 μl./ml. After incubation of unwashed ova with unwashed spermatozoa (under 5% CO_2 in air), the O_2 content was 3.27 μl./ml. The O_2 content after incubation of unwashed ova with centrifuged spermatozoa, that were resuspended in the solution used for sperm recovery, was 3.18 μl. O_2/ml. The O_2 content of the defined medium containing the capacitators' ova was 2.99 μl. O_2/ml. at the same time.

DISCUSSION

This investigation revealed that by washing the uterine spermatozoa something happens to the sperm cells which decreases their ability to fertilize ova in vitro. It was thought that this effect might be caused by removal from the sperm cells of some soluble substance which was carried into the fertilization medium by spermatozoa from the uterine environment of the capacitator. Since enhancement of the fertilization of washed ova by washed spermatozoa could not be accomplished by adding sperm washings back to the washed sperm cells, it is concluded that if a substance was removed from the spermatozoa by the washing procedure, the substance was very labile. This idea is further substantiated by the experiments in which ampullary oviduct fluid was used.

An alternative explanation for these results lies in the fact that the composition of the atmosphere was not controlled throughout the sperm-washing procedure. The effect on the spermatozoa could very well be due to an alteration of CO_2 or O_2 tension in the vicinity of the sperm cells during the washing procedure. A reduced O_2 tension favors fertilization in vitro. The O_2 contents of the fertilization mediums ranged from 2.49 to 3.27 μl. $O_2/ml.$, or approximately 9–12% O_2. These values were slightly higher than those reported for O_2 content in the rabbit oviduct,[3, 16] but were compatible with the fertilization process in Experiment 15-110-I (Table 4).

In most of the experiments of this investigation, the initial gamete incubation was under an air atmosphere. It was rediscovered that a moist 5% CO_2 in air atmosphere is beneficial to in-vitro fertilization and early development. The fact that the gametes were initially incubated under a moist 5% CO_2 in air atmosphere in previous work[5] was overlooked because the tightly sealed Carrel flasks used were thought to be isolated from any influence of the gas content of the surrounding atmosphere. In this investigation, the increased CO_2 influenced events inside the sealable tissue culture dishes even though all air space above the fertilization medium was filled with paraffin oil, and the thin layer of oil between ground glass surfaces of the dishes made an apparent seal.

Thibault and Dauzier found that washing the ova prior to incubation with capacitated spermatozoa was beneficial to their in-vitro fertilization results.[20, 21] They postulated that a substance, "fertilizin," was removed from the ova by the in-vitro washing procedure, or by an "antifertilizin" in vivo. Bedford and Chang found that no benefit was gained by washing the ova in their experiments. The slight increase in the proportion of ova fertilized following washing in this work was not statistically significant.

Brinster reported that the optimum osmolarity for in-vitro culture of mouse ova was 276 mosm.[6] This value is close to those measured in this work for oviduct fluid—272 mosm., and rabbit serum—279 mosm. The 345 milliosmolar-defined medium was probably not so good an environment for fertilization as the 280 milliosmolar medium. The 287 milliosmolar 10% serum solution was far superior to the 221 milliosmolar solution for ovum culture.

The impression was gained that better results were obtained when the capacitators were not given injections of HCG or when they were given injections of only 50 I.U. than when they were given 75 I.U. HCG. Soupart has reported that fertilization in vivo was markedly reduced when capacitators were given more than 75 I.U. HCG.[18] The effect of HCG on fertilization by capacitated spermatozoa in vitro may be similar to that found in vivo.

Barros and Austin have fertilized hamster ova in vitro, using ova removed from ovarian follicles and spermatozoa, and from the cauda epididymis of mature males. In this way, they avoided any role the uterus or oviduct might normally play in the fertilization process or in preparing the gametes for fertilization. A step in this direction has been taken in the present work. Fertilization of rabbit ova can take place in the absence of secretions from the female reproductive tract. However, the conditions which allow rabbit ova and spermatozoa to unite without any prior conditioning influences by the female reproductive tract remain for future investigation.

SUMMARY

In-vitro fertilization experiments were carried out to assess the effects of washing the secretions of the female reproductive tract from rabbit ova and spermatozoa prior to their incubation together. Ova from each ovum donor and capacitated spermatozoa from each capacitator were divided into approximately equal parts. Half the ova was incubated in vitro with half the spermatozoa after washing one or both types of gametes, while the other half of the ova was incubated in vitro with the other half of the spermatozoa after washing both types of gametes, or after no special washing of either type of gamete. The proportions of ova fertilized in each case were compared.

Washing both ova and spermatozoa caused a statistically significant decrease in the proportion of ova that could be fertilized in vitro when neither type gamete was washed. This decrease was accounted for by washing only the spermatozoa. Neither washings of uterine spermatozoa from previous experiments, nor ampullary oviduct fluid, when added back to washed spermatozoa, were able to restore the fertilizing ability to a level expected for unwashed spermatozoa. The possible explanations for this result are: (1) an extremely labile soluble substance from the uterine environment was removed from the sperm cells by washing, or (2) the O_2 and/or CO_2 tensions were changed in the vicinity of the sperm cells during the experimental procedure.

REFERENCES

1. BARROS, C., and AUSTIN, C. R.   In vitro fertilization of golden hamster ova. Anat Rec 157:209, 1967.
2. BEDFORD, J. M., and CHANG, M. C.   Fertilization of rabbit ova in vitro. Nature (London) 193:898, 1962.
3. BISHOP, D. W.   Oxygen concentrations in the rabbit genital tract. Int Congr Anim Reprod 3:53, 1956.
4. BRACKETT, B. G., and WILLIAMS, W. L.   In vitro fertilization of rabbit ova. J Exp Zool 160:271, 1965.

5. BRACKETT, B. G., and WILLIAMS, W. L.   Fertilization of rabbit ova in a defined medium. *Fertil Steril 19*:144, 1968.
6. BRINSTER, R. L.   Studies on the development of mouse embryos *in vitro*. I. The effect of osmolarity and hydrogen ion concentration. *J Exp Zool 158*:49, 1965.
7. BRINSTER, R. L.   Lactate dehydrogenase activity in the pre-implantation rabbit embryo. *Biochim Biophys Acta 148*:298, 1967.
8. CHANG, M. C.   Fertilization of rabbit ova *in vitro. Nature (London) 184*:466, 1959.
9. DAUZIER, L., and THIBAULT, C.   Recherches expérimentale sur la maturation des gametes male chez les mammifères, par l'étude de la fecondation "in vitro" de l'oeuf de lapine. *Proceedings, IIIrd International Congress on Animal Reproduction, Cambridge,* 1956, Sect. I, p. 58.
10. DAUZIER, L., and THIBAULT, C.   Donnees nouvelles sur la fecondation *in vitro* de l'oeuf de la lapine et de la Brebis. *C R Acad Sci 248*:2655, 1959.
11. DAUZIER, L., and THIBAULT, C.   La fecondation *in vitro* de l'oeuf de lapine. *Proceedings, IVth International Congress on Animal Reproduction, The Hague,* 1961, p. 727.
12. DAUZIER, L., THIBAULT, C., and WINTENBERGER, S.   La fecondation in vitro de l'oeuf de la lapine. *C R Acad Sci (Paris) 238*:844, 1954.
13. DAVID, A., BRACKETT, B. G., GARCIA, C-R., and MASTROIANNI, L.   Composition of rabbit segmental oviduct fluid. *J Reprod Fertil* (In press)
14. MORICARD, R.   Observation of *in vitro* fertilization in the rabbit. *Nature (London) 173*:1140, 1954.
15. MORICARD, R.   Penetration spermatique obtenue *in vitro* au travers de la membrane pellucide d'ovocytes de lapine cultives dans les liquides de secretion uterotubaire. *C R Soc Biol (Paris) 148*:423, 1954.
16. MASTROIANNI, L., and JONES, R.   Oxygen tension within the rabbit fallopian tube. *J Reprod Fertil 9*:99, 1965.
17. SMITH, A. U.   Fertilization *in vitro* of the mammalian egg: The biochemistry of fertilization and the gametes. *Biochem Soc Symp 7*:3, 1951.
18. SOUPART, P.   Effects of HCG on capacitation of rabbit spermatozoa. *Nature (London) 212*:408, 1966.
19. SUZUKI, SHUETU, and MASTROIANNI, LUIGI, JR.   *In vitro* fertilization of rabbit ova in tubal fluid. *Amer J Obstet Gynec 93*:465, 1965.
20. THIBAULT, C., and DAUZIER, L.   "Fertilisines" et fecondation *in vitro* de l'oeuf de lapine. *C R Acad Sci (Paris) 250*:1358, 1960.
21. THIBAULT, C., and DAUZIER, L.   Analyse des conditions de la fecondation *in vitro* de l'oeuf de la lapine. *Ann Biol Anim Biochem Biophys 1*:277, 1961.
22. THIBAULT, C., DAUZIER, L., and WINTENBERGER, S.   Etude cytologique de la fecondation *in vitro* de l'oeuf de la lapine. *C R Soc Biol (Paris) 148*:789, 1954.
23. WILLIAMS, W. L., HAMNER, C. E., WEINMAN, D. E., and BRACKETT, B. G.   Capacitation of rabbit spermatozoa and initial experiments on *in vitro* fertilization. *Proceedings Vth International Congress on Animal Reproduction, Trento,* 1964, Sect. VII, p. 288.

IN VITRO FERTILIZATION OF RABBIT OVA: TIME SEQUENCE OF EVENTS[*]

BENJAMIN G. BRACKETT, D.V.M., Ph.D.

The sequence of events in fertilization, from sperm penetration to zygote cleavage, and their time relationships are well-known for ova of several mammalian species. The fertilization process in the rabbit has been studied by many investigators. The purpose of the present investigation was to observe the development of the fertilization process of the rabbit in vitro and to compare these observations on in vitro fertilization with those previously made on in vivo fertilization.

MATERIALS AND METHODS

In vitro fertilization of rabbit ova was carried out by the best procedure reported previously.[4] Mature New Zealand White does were used after an isolation period of at least 19 days. Ovum donors were superovulated, in the way described previously, with 50 I.U. of Human Chorionic Gonadotropin (A.P.L., Ayerst Labs., New York, N. Y.) being used as the ovulating dose. The sperm capacitators were also injected with 50 I.U. of Human Chorionic Gonadotropin at the time of mating.

Ova from the same donors were incubated with spermatozoa recovered from the same capacitator in each experiment, i.e., each of two tissue culture dishes contained gametes which came from the same sources. One group of ova, in the experimental dish, was removed from the incubator at a different time from the other

* Supported by Grants FR00340-03 and HDO-1810-04A1 from the National Institutes of Health, United States Public Health Service, and by the Ford Foundation.

group of ova, in the control dish. By comparing the proportion of ova at a certain stage in the fertilization process with the proportion of control ova that were normally cleaved at 24–26 hr. postinsemination, it was possible to evaluate the completion of certain stages of the fertilization process in vitro. The events studied in this way were the penetration of capacitated spermatozoa through the zona pellucida and the formation of pronuclei. Penetration of the vitellus by a spermatozoon was observed on one occasion, and cleavage of in vitro fertilized ova was observed on several occasions. The later stages of fertilization, i.e., pronuclei and syngamy, as well as early cleavages, were also observed in ova that were fertilized in vivo.

These observations were made by phase-contrast microscopy and time-lapse microcinematography. Ova were either examined and photographed on a microscope slide, compressed under a cover glass at room temperature, or, for observations of cleavage, were held at 37° C. in a small Embdeco perfusion chamber (Coleman Instruments, Inc., Maywood, Ill.) under an air curtain incubator (Sage Laboratories, Inc., New York, N. Y.). Time-lapse pictures were taken at 16 frames/min. on 16-mm. film under phase contrast.

RESULTS

Sperm Penetration of the Zona Pellucida. In experiments in which ova were removed from the 5% CO_2 in air atmosphere at 2–2¼ hr. after insemination in vitro, very vigorously motile spermatozoa were only occasionally seen within the perivitelline space. A surrounding layer of corona radiata cells made the detection of one or more sperm cells inside the perivitelline space dependent on the observation of the motility of the sperm cells and of the vitellus itself. That sperm penetration had occurred could be convincingly documented only by time-lapse photography. Three of 16 ova (19%) were penetrated by at least one sperm cell when examined 2–2¼ hr. after insemination in vitro, whereas 12 of 18 in vitro fertilized control ova (67%) cleaved normally.

By 3 hr. postinsemination, all of the ova that were to be fertilized in vitro had been penetrated by at least one sperm cell. This conclusion was drawn from data shown in Table 1. Although the fertilization rate was lower than usual in these experiments, it is obvious that the same proportion of ova in experimental dishes were penetrated as the proportion of ova that cleaved normally in the control dishes. Of the 18 in vitro fertilized control ova, 15 were in the 4-cell stage, and 3 were in the 2-cell stage.

Penetration of the Vitellus by a Spermatozoon. On one occasion, a sperm cell was observed to penetrate the vitellus. This ovum was removed from the CO_2 incubator and placed on a slide at room temperature approximately 3 hr. postinsemination. Time-lapse pictures were begun at 3 hr. 50 min. postinsemination. One very actively motile sperm cell was seen inside the perivitelline space, and it was vigorously swimming and bumping into the comparatively rigid zona pellucida, as has

been frequently observed in ova examined at this time. At approximately 4 hr. 10 min. postinsemination, the sperm cell appeared to change directions in order to stick onto the vitelline surface. The sperm tail remained actively motile throughout the penetration process, which occurred gradually over a period of approximately 23 min. (Fig. 1). The sperm tail followed the head into the vitellus. Some activity could be seen on the movie film immediately following the complete disappearance of the sperm cell from the perivitelline space, but the thickness of the vitellus made development into a male pronucleus impossible to observe under the conditions used.

Formation of Pronuclei. Male pronuclei were observed in ova undergoing fertilization in vitro as early as 4 hr. after insemination. Four of 8 ova had a male pronucleus at 4 hr., and 1 of the 2 control ova was in the 4-cell stage at 24 hr. postinsemination. Pronuclear development was observed and, by 9 hr postinsemination, both male and female pronuclei were well-formed.

Data from observations made between 6½ and 9 hr. postinsemination are shown in Table 2. In Experiment 18-94, all 4 ova that were undergoing fertilization had 2 polar bodies, and 1 had very motile spermatozoa inside the perivitelline space. In 1 of these ova the pronuclei were already in juxtaposition. At 6½ hr. (Experiment 21-19-II), male pronuclei could be seen as lighter areas within the vitellus under low magnification (15×). The development of pronuclei was continuously observed in one of these ova. By 8¼ hr. postinsemination, in this ovum, both male and female pronuclei were well-defined entities as seen under phase contrast. Of the 24 in vitro fertilized control ova observed 26 hr. after insemination, 4 were in the 8-cell, 16 were in the 4-cell, and 5 were in the 2-cell stage.

In Experiments 18-94 and 20-3, and in the following 2 experiments in which cleavage was observed, the capacitated sperma-

TABLE 1. *Observation of Penetrated and Cleaved Ova at Intervals Following Insemination in Vitro*

Exp. no.	No. of ova penetrated/ova recovered after 3 hr.	No. of ova cleaved/ova recovered after 24 hr.
18-73	1/4	2/8
20-51	6/25	3/23
20-69	2/9	7/12
21-10	6/10	4/5
21-40	2/6	2/6
Summary	17/54 (31.5%)	18/54 (33.3%)

48

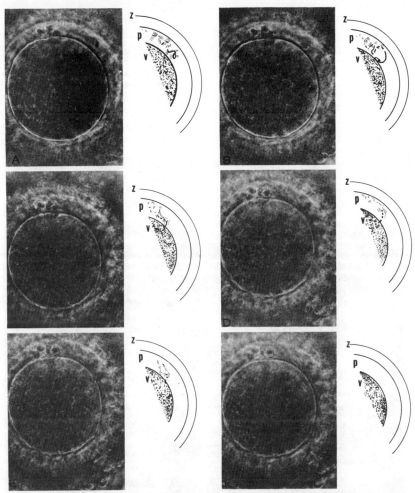

Fig. 1. Penetration of the vitellus by a spermatozoon. The sperm cell appears in the photographs at 1 o'clock. z, zona pellucida; p, perivitelline space; v, vitellus. A, 4 hr. 10 min postinsemination. A single sperm cell is freely swimming in the perivitelline space; B, 4 hr. 13 min. postinsemination. The sperm head is stuck on the vitellus; C, 4 hr. 18 min. postinsemination. The sperm head has entered the vitellus; D, 4 hr. 26 min. postinsemination. The motile sperm tail is observed in the perivitelline space; E, 4 hr. 29 min. postinsemination. Part of the tail is still visible in the perivitelline space; F, 4 hr. 35 min. postinsemination. The sperm cell has completely penetrated into the vitellus.

tozoa used were recovered 18 hr. after mating with the capacitator doe, in contrast to the usual 13-hr. interval.

Cleavage. In an experiment in which the experimental ova were examined 15 hr. 50 min. after insemination, 12 of 15 ova (80%) provided evidence of undergoing fertilization. Two ova were already in the

49

TABLE 2. *Observations of Pronuclear State and Cleaved Ova at Intervals Following Insemination in Vitro*

Exp. no.	No. of ova in pronuclear stage/ova recovered after 6½–9 hr.	No. of ova cleaved/ova recovered after 26 hr.
18-94	4/6	10/15
20-3	4/4	6/8
21-19-II	7/9	8/12 .
Totals	15/19 (79%)	24/35 (69%)

2-cell stage; cleavage was estimated to have begun approximately 20 min. before. Three ova were in the process of cleaving. Five ova were in the pronuclear stage. One ovum had 2 polar bodies, and another had at least 1 actively motile sperm cell inside the perivitelline space. Seven of 14 in vitro fertilized control ova (50%) cleaved. Five were in the 8-cell stage and 2 were in the 2-cell stage at 28 hr. postinsemination.

One ovum which was examined 15 hr. 40 min. after insemination contained pronuclei which were undergoing syngamy. The pronuclei disappeared at approximately 17 hr. postinsemination, and cleavage occurred in a span of 5–8 min., a ½-hr. afterward. This sequence of events is shown in Fig. 2. Later cleavages of in vitro fertilized ova to 10–12 cells, as well as cleavages of in vivo fertilized ova, have been observed. Each blastomere under-

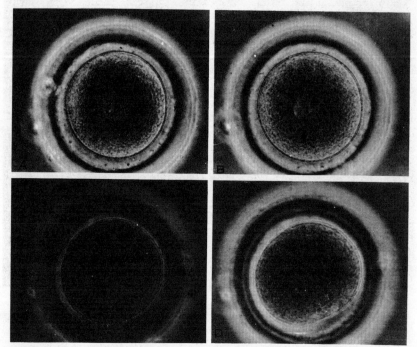

FIG. 2. Syngamy and cleavage of an in vitro fertilized ovum. *A*, 16 hr. 45 min. postinsemination. Pronuclei are undergoing syngamy; *B*, 16 hr. 55 min. postinsemination. Pronuclei are losing their identity; *C*, 17 hr. 40 min. postinsemination. Vitellus is becoming flattened; *D*, 17 hr. 41 min. postinsemination. Vitellus is definitely flattened; *E*, 17 hr. 43 min. postinsemination. Indentation is apparent; *F*, 17 hr. 44 min. postinsemination. Cleavage is underway; *G*, 17 hr. 45 min. postinsemination. Cleavage is underway; *H*, 17 hr. 46 min. postinsemination. Cleavage appears to be complete; *I*, 17 hr. 48 min. postinsemination. Two-cell stage ovum.

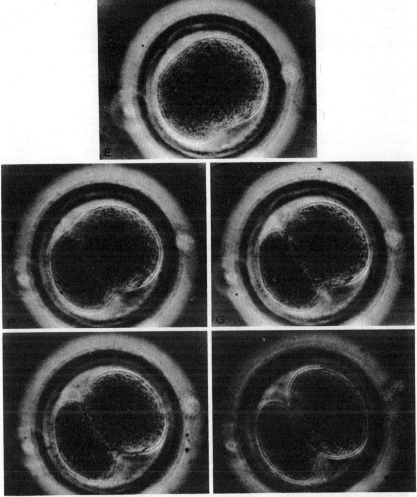

FIG. 2—Continued

going division was seen to divide completely in less than 10 min.

The first cleavage was observed in one other in vitro fertilization experiment in which at least 3 of 30 ova were in the 2-cell stage, 15½ hr. after insemination. Cleavage of the 4-cell stage was first observed at 18½ hr. after insemination, and in vitro fertilized ova were found in the 8-cell stage as early as 26 hr. postinsemination.

In each of 2 experiments, ova from one dish were examined at 24 hr. postinsemination while ova from the other dish were

51

transferred to fresh 10% serum solution at 24 hr.[5] and examined at 48 hr. postinsemination. At 24 hr. postinsemination, 17 of 45 ova (38%) had cleaved. Fourteen were in the 4-cell stage, and 3 were in the 2-cell stage. At 48 hr. postinsemination, 14 of 30 ova (47%) were in various cleavage stages. Six were in at least the 16-cell (morula) stage, 4 were in the 8-cell stage, 1 was in the 4-cell stage, and 3 were in the 2-cell stage. Therefore, 6 of 14 in vitro fertilized ova (43%) developed to the morula stage in culture.

DISCUSSION

Sperm penetration in the rabbit occurs 10–13 hr. postcoitus with most of the ova being penetrated in the 1st hr. after ovulation.[3, 12] In the present study, sperm penetration was also complete by 3 hr., but most of the ova were penetrated between 2 and 3 hr. after exposure of the ova to capacitated spermatozoa. According to Thibault and Dauzier approximately 2 hr. is required for the dispersal from the ovum surface of a substance that prevents capacitated spermatozoa from sticking to the zona pellucida.[15]

In agreement with reported observations in the rat[1] and hamster,[16] I gained the impression that the motility of the sperm cell was not the only force at work in penetration of the vitellus, although the sperm tail did maintain its motility as long as it was visible in the perivitelline space. The entire sperm cell, including the tail, penetrated the vitellus. No swelling was seen in the area of the vitellus that was penetrated, but the observation reported here cannot deny the existence of such a feature, since the sperm cell may not have been exactly at the periphery of the vitellus when penetration occurred. Penetration of the vitellus may take place very rapidly after penetration of the zona pellucida in vivo, as has been suggested in previous work,[1, 16] but the observations reported here indicate that rabbit spermatozoa can remain motile

for long periods in the perivitelline space and penetration of the vitellus may begin to occur at room temperature at a time 20 min. or longer after penetration of the zona pellucida.

Second polar body formation occurs 13–14½ hr. postcoitus, and male pronucleus formation occurs between 14 and 18 hr. postcoitus in the rabbit.[7, 11] These events were observed to take place in a comparable time in the present in vitro fertilization experiments, when allowance is made for the slower time of sperm penetration.

The first cleavage of fertilized rabbit ova normally occurs 21–25 hr. postcoitus, or roughly 11–15 hr. after exposure of ova to capacitated spermatozoa in vivo.[8, 11] Cleavage to the 4-cell stage occurs 25–32 hr. postcoitus. Cleavage to the 8-cell and 16-cell stages occurs 32–40 hr. and 40–47 hr. postcoitus, respectively.[2, 9]

The earliest observed cleavage to the 2-cell stage was 15½ hr. after in vitro insemination. A range of time spent in each cleavage stage could not accurately be determined, since some ova failed to cleave more than once after fertilization in vitro. However, I gained the impression throughout this and previous studies[4-6] that the duration of the cleavage stages in vitro is comparable to the duration of those in vivo. It is interesting that live young have developed following the surgical transfer of in vitro fertilized rabbit ova when the cleavage stages were definitely delayed[13] as well as when the cleavage stages were the same as would have been present in vivo.[4] Development of 43% of in vitro fertilized ova to the morula stage in culture compares favorably with the 22% development reported by Suzuki.[14]

Microcinematography has been employed by Moricard in a previous study of fertilization of rabbit ova in vivo and in vitro.[10] This method was proposed as a means of documenting the presence of actively motile spermatozoa within the perivitelline space, and such an observation was suggested as a test for the first stage of fertilization in the rabbit. Moricard studied in vivo penetrated ova in this manner. Similar observations of in vitro penetrated ova have been made in the present study, and the author concludes that such observations provide an excellent in vitro assay for the ability of spermatozoa to penetrate the zona pellucida (sperm capacitation).

Lewis and Gregory were the first to employ microcinematography in observations on cleavage stages of in vivo fertilized rabbit ova.[9] Similar observations of cleavage have been made in the author's laboratory, and it is concluded that in vitro fertilized ova develop in a comparable manner to those fertilized in vivo.

SUMMARY

Observations were made on fertilization of rabbit ova in vitro by phase-contrast microscopy and time-lapse microcinematography. It was found that sperm penetration through the zona pellucida was complete by 3 hr. after exposure of the ova to capacitated spermatozoa. Male and female pronuclei were fully developed by 9 hr. after insemination. In vitro fertilized ova cleaved to the 2-, 4-, and 8-cell stages as early as 15½, 18½, and 26 hr. postinsemination, respectively. Some ova developed to the morula stage by 48 hr. postinsemination.

Penetration of the vitellus of one ovum by a sperm cell was observed and documented by time-lapse microcinematography. The sperm cell remained free in the perivitelline space for at least 20 min. before sticking to the vitelline membrane. The entire sperm cell entered the vitellus over an interval of approximately 23 min. at room temperature.

Cleavage of in vitro fertilized ova was observed on several occasions. The cleavage process was shown to occur over a span of 5–8 min. No difference could be seen in the sequence of events of fertilization and early cleavage between rabbit ova fertilized in vivo and rabbit ova fertilized in vitro.

Acknowledgments. The author gratefully acknowledges the technical assistance of Mrs. Eva Kelly, Miss Stefanie Shattuck, and Mr. Don Killen.

REFERENCES

1. AUSTIN, C. R. Observations on the penetration of sperm into the mammalian egg. *Aust J Sci Res B 4:*581, 1951.
2. AUSTIN, C. R. "Fertilization and Transport of the Ovum." In *Conference on Physiological Mechanisms Concerned with Conception.* Pergamon, New York, 1963, p. 285.
3. AUSTIN, C. R., AND BRADEN, A. W. H. Time relations and their significance in the ovulation and penetration of eggs in rats and rabbit. *Aust J Biol Sci 7:*179, 1954.
4. BRACKETT, B. G. Effects of washing the gametes on fertilization in vitro. *Fertil Steril 20:*127, 1969.
5. BRACKETT, B. G., AND WILLIAMS, W. L. In vitro fertilization of rabbit ova. *J Exp Zool 160:* 271, 1965.
6. BRACKETT, B. G., AND WILLIAMS, W. L. Fertilization of rabbit ova in a defined medium. *Fertil Steril 19:*144, 1968.
7. CHANG, M. C. Fertility and sterility as revealed in the study of fertilization and development of rabbit eggs. *Fertil Steril 2:*205, 1951.
8. CHANG, M. C. Fertilization of domestic rabbit (Oryctolagus cuniculus) ova by cottontail rabbit (Sylvilagus transitionalis) sperm. *J Exp Zool 144:*1, 1960.
9. LEWIS, W. H., AND GREGORY, P. W. Cinematographs of living developing rabbit eggs. *Science 69:*226, 1929.
10. MORICARD, R. Observations of in vitro fertilization in the rabbit. *Nature 173:*1140, 1954.
11. PINCUS, G. The comparative behavior of mammalian eggs in vivo and in vitro. IV. The development of fertilized and artificially activated rabbit eggs. *J Exp Zool 82:*85, 1939.
12. PINCUS, G., AND ENZMANN, E. V. Fertilization in the rabbit. *J Exp Biol 9:*403, 1932.
13. SEITZ, H. M., JR., BRACKETT, B. G., AND MASTROIANNI, L., JR. In vitro fertilization of ovulated rabbit ova recovered from the ovary. Submitted for publication.

14. Suzuki, S. In vitro cultivation of rabbit ova following in vitro fertilization in tubal fluid. *Cytologia 31*:416, 1966.

15. Thibault, C., and Dauzier, L. Analyse des conditions de la fécondation in vitro de l'oeuf de là lapine. *Ann Biol Anim Biochem Biophys 1*:27, 1961.

16. Yanagimachi, R. Time and process of sperm penetration into hamster ova in vivo and in vitro. *J Reprod Fertil 11*:359, 1966.

72968

T. Iwamatsu
M. C. Chang

In vitro Fertilization of Mouse Eggs in the Presence of Bovine Follicular Fluid

SINCE the recognition of "capacitation of sperm" in the female tract[1,2], fertilization *in vitro* of eggs has been successfully conducted by insemination of sperm recovered from the uterus for the rabbit[3,4], hamster[5] and mouse[6]. Successful fertilization of golden hamster eggs *in vitro* by epididymal (uncapacitated) hamster sperm[5], in the presence of follicular fluid of hamster[7] or cow[8], or in the presence of rabbit tubal cyst fluid (our unpublished work), and that of Chinese hamster eggs in the presence of follicular fluid of golden hamster[9], encouraged us to carry out the following experiment which demonstrated that mouse sperm can be capacitated *in vitro* to fertilize mouse eggs in the presence of bovine follicular fluid.

Female Swiss–Webster mice, weighing 21–24 g, were superovulated by intraperitoneal injection of 5 IU of pregnant mare serum in 0·1 ml. of saline (Equinex, Ayerst Lab.) and 5 IU of human chorionic gonadotrophin (HCG) in 0·1 ml. of saline (APL, Ayerst Lab.) 48 h later. They were killed 14–16 h after injection of HCG and their eggs were recovered under extra heavy mineral oil in a watch glass, according to the description of Yanagimachi and Chang[5]. Sperm suspension was prepared by mincing a cauda epididymis in a watch glass containing 1 ml. of warm Tyrode solution (Difco) supplemented with 100 IU/ml. of penicillin G and 50 µg/ml. of streptomycin sulphate. Fluid was collected from large follicles of cow ovaries obtained from a slaughter house, and from human ovaries obtained from a hospital. Follicular fluid was withdrawn with a syringe to avoid contamination of blood, kept in a test tube and stored in a refrigerator (at 0°–5° C). The fluid was used within 2 weeks of collection. Fluid was collected in the same way from tubal cysts of rabbit and cow, stored and used within 3 days.

At the time of insemination three drops (about 0·03 ml.) of sperm suspension were taken up in a fine glass pipette (about 100 microns in diameter) and added to the egg clot under mineral oil. Two drops of the suspension were added to the other egg clot to which one drop (about 0·01 ml.) of heated bovine or human follicular fluid, or tubal cyst fluid of rabbit or cow, had already been added. In some cases the egg clot was washed three times by transferring it into 0·5 ml. of warm Tyrode solution covered with mineral oil. After insemination the preparation was thoroughly mixed by means of a glass needle and incubated at 37° C in an atmosphere of 5 per cent carbon dioxide and 95 per cent oxygen for 1–6 h. The final count in each watch glass was 8,000–14,000 sperm mm[3].

At the end of the period of incubation the proportions of motile sperm and sperm with (Fig. 1*a*) or without

(Fig. 1b) acrosomes were determined. A drop of suspension was taken from each preparation, mixed with an equal volume of saline containing 2 per cent egg white (to slow down motility), covered with a cover slip and examined under a phase-contrast microscope. After counting the eggs were washed in saline, placed on a slide in the centre of four spots of vaseline, compressed carefully under a cover slip, and examined under phase-contrast for evidence of sperm penetration. Eggs were considered to have been penetrated only when there was an enlarged sperm head or a male pronucleus in the vitellus with fertilizing sperm tail in or around the vitellus.

The proportion of motile sperm, with and without acrosomes, at any time between 1 and 6 h after insemination varied from 43 per cent to 64 per cent in any preparation. The pattern of motility appeared to be different between those with an acrosome (intact sperm) and those without (reacted sperm). In the intact sperm the midpiece was sharply bent during movement. Sperm without an acrosome were propelled by a wave of beats from the midpiece to the tip of the tail. Although numerous sperm were attached to the zona pellucida within 15 min of

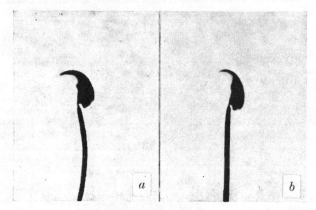

Fig. 1. *a*, Intact mouse sperm with acrosome; *b*, reacted mouse sperm without acrosome (× 2,200).

insemination, the detachment of the acrosome and its penetration through the zona was not observed less than 2 h after insemination. Obviously in our experimental condition mouse epididymal sperm need at least about 2 h for capacitation. It has been reported that capacitation of mouse sperm in the female tract may be unnecessary or require only 1 h (ref. 10). Apparently the process of sperm capacitation takes longer *in vitro* than *in vivo*.

Table 1 reveals some interesting facts. In the presence of the bovine follicular fluid the proportion of motile sperm without acrosomes increased from 7·6 per cent 2 h after insemination to 28 per cent after 6 h. This increase correlated approximately with the proportion of eggs

Table 1. *In vitro* FERTILIZATION OF MOUSE EGGS IN THE PRESENCE OF BOVINE FOLLICULAR FLUID

Media	Incubation time (h)	Percentage of motile sperm without acrosome (means)	No. of eggs	Total (per cent)	Monospermic	Polyspermic
Tyrode solution with	1	0	200	0	0	0
half volume of bovine	2	7·6	240	1 (0·4)	1	0
follicular fluid	3	14·2	288	51 (17·7)	38	13
Heated at 60° C for	4	14·2	278	100 (35·9)	52	48
10 min	5	21·0	195	72 (36·9)	34	38
	6	28·0	225	75 (33·3)	49	26
Tyrode solution	1	0·4	213	0	0	0
	2	0·7	167	2 (1·2)	0	2
	3	2·7	196	13 (6·6)	7	6
	4	12·6	268	29 (10·8)	26	3
	5	13·6	223	49 (21·9)	33	16
Tyrode solution, egg clot	1	0	111	0	0	0
washed three times	2	1·5	101	0	0	0
	3	5·1	115	1 (0·9)	1	0
	4	3·0	137	2 (1·4)	2	0
	5	5·8	112	20 (17·8)	10	10
Tyrode solution with half	4	—	219	22 (10·0)	12	10
volume of rabbit tube-	7	—	92	13 (14·1)	11	2
cyst fluid	10*	—	57	15 (26·3)	12	3
Unheated						
Tyrode solution with half	4	—	132	13 (9·8)	7	6
volume of bovine tube-						
cyst fluid						
Heated at 55° C for						
10 min						
Tyrode solution with half	4	—	169	16 (10·8)	12	4
volume of human fol-						
licular fluid						
Heated at 70° C for						
10 min						

* Sperm were incubated for 4 h before insemination.

penetrated. Although the proportion of motile sperm without acrosomes increased slightly, from 14·2 per cent after 4 h to 28 per cent after 6 h, the proportion of eggs penetrated did not increase between 4 h (35·9 per cent) to 6 h after insemination (33·3 per cent). This may indicate that either the proportion of capacitated sperm was insufficient to penetrate many eggs or that the physiological integrity of sperm and eggs declined 4 h after insemination. Nevertheless, the proportion of eggs penetrated (37 per cent) by epididymal sperm in our experimental condition is not significantly less than the best results obtained by Whittingham (41 per cent) with uterine sperm[6].

In the absence of bovine follicular fluid, and especially after the egg clot had been washed in Tyrode solution, the proportions of active sperm without an acrosome and of penetrated eggs increased only slightly between 2 and 5 h after insemination. There was a significant difference ($P < 0.001$) in the proportion of eggs that had been penetrated 4 h after insemination between preparations with and without bovine follicular fluid, and also between preparations which were washed or not, and so we conclude that bovine follicular fluid has a beneficial effect on the capacitation of mouse sperm. Washing the egg clot in Tyrode solution could remove some factor that is beneficial to capacitation and fertilization *in vitro*. In the presence of fluid from tubal cysts of rabbits or cows and of human follicular fluid, the proportion of penetrated eggs 4 or 7 h after insemination (9·8–14·1 per cent) was not significantly greater than in Tyrode solution (10·8 per cent). This indicates that the beneficial factor is in a higher concentration in the bovine follicular fluid than in the other fluids. As in the case of *in vitro* fertilization of hamster eggs[5], the proportion of polyspermic eggs was high compared with *in vivo* conditions[10]. Many of the penetrated eggs cleaved when cultured, and it is likely most of them had been truly fertilized.

The elevation and loss of the acrosome in the female tract of many rodent sperm have been considered to constitute "capacitation"[11]. When hamster eggs were inseminated with epididymal sperm in the presence of hamster follicular fluid the acrosome reaction occurred and a high proportion of eggs were fertilized *in vitro*[7]. When hamster epididymal sperm were incubated in the presence of hamster follicular fluid they lost their acrosome, were extremely motile and penetrated eggs as early as 10 min after insemination *in vitro*[12]. Heated bovine follicular fluid has been reported to contain two factors responsible for the induction of the acrosome reaction and capacitation of hamster sperm[8]. Although one factor is known to be dialysable and heat stable, while the other is non-dialysable and heat labile[8], how these two factors interact to achieve capacitation leading to penetration has yet to be determined. The work reported here, however, has shown that the acrosome reaction of mouse epididymal sperm can be induced, and the capacitation of mouse sperm can be achieved *in vitro* in the presence of heated bovine follicular fluid.

This work was supported by grants from the Ford Foundation and the US Public Health Service. We thank Dr H. W. Horne for the human ovaries and Mrs Rose Bartke for technical assistance.

[1] Austin, C. R., *Austral. J. Sci. Res.*, Series B, Biol. Sci., **4**, 581 (1951).
[2] Chang, M. C., *Nature*, **168**, 697 (1951).
[3] Thibault, C., Dauzier, L., and Wintenberger, S., *CR Soc. Biol.*, **148**, 789 (1954).
[4] Chang, M. C., *Nature*, **184**, 466 (1959).
[5] Yanagimachi, R., and Chang, M. C., *Nature*, **200**, 281 (1963).
[6] Whittingham, D. G., *Nature*, **220**, 592 (1968).
[7] Barros, C., and Austin, C. R., *J. Exp. Zool.*, **166**, 317 (1967).
[8] Yanagimachi, R., *J. Exp. Zool.*, **170**, 269 (1969).
[9] Pickworth, S., and Chang, M. C., *J. Reprod. Fert.*, **19**, 371 (1969).
[10] Braden, A. W. H., and Austin, C. R., *Austral. J. Biol. Sci.*, 7, 552 (1954).
[11] Austin, C. R., and Bishop, M. W. H., *Proc. Roy. Soc.*, B, **149**, 241 (1958).
[12] Yanagimachi, R., *J. Reprod. Fert.*, **18**, 275 (1969).

IN VITRO FERTILIZATION OF MAMMALIAN EGGS

M. C. CHANG [1]

THE literature on the fertilization *in vitro* of mammalian eggs has been reviewed by many workers (Chang and Pincus, 1951; Smith, 1951; Austin, 1951, 1961; Austin and Bishop, 1957; Chang, 1957; Thibault and Dauzier, 1961.) The experiments designed to obtain the fertilization of mammalian eggs *in vitro* from 1878 (Schenk, 1878) to 1959 (Chang, 1959) listed by Austin (1961), encompass 35 papers by 21 authors from different countries. Although "uterine eggs" of guinea pigs and rabbits were used in one case (Onanoff, 1893), the tubal eggs of rabbits and to a lesser extent the follicular eggs of humans have been used most commonly. According to this table, the sperm used were either ejaculated or epididymal, but sperm from the uterus were used only in the more recent studies which followed the discovery of the need for capacitation as a pre-requisite for fertilization (Austin, 1951; Chang, 1951). As for the criteria of fertilization, sperm entry into the egg, emission of the second polar body, shrinkage of the vitellus, formation of pronuclei and cleavage were considered as evidence of fertilization in most studies. Although the birth of young has been reported in three investigations (Pincus and Enzmann, 1934; Venge, 1953; Chang, 1959) in which eggs fertilized *in vitro* were transferred into foster mothers, Austin (1961) considered that the best supported case for fertilization *in vitro* was done by Chang (1959).

Due to the technical difficulties involved in conducting such experiments and lack of confirmation of these experiments by others, together with the unreliability of the criteria of fertilization used by some investigators, the evidence for fertilization of mammalian eggs *in vitro* even at present may be still in doubt, and it becomes to some extent a controversial issue.

In the early studies of fertilization either *in vivo* or *in vitro*, most investigators considered fertilization to mean the penetration of a sperm into the cytoplasm of the egg, but in reality this phase is only the beginning of fertilization. Biologically, fertilization is a physiological process, which starts with the penetration of sperm into the cytoplasm of the egg, and includes the subsequent formation, development and syngamy of the male and female pronuclei until the union of maternal and paternal genetic materials. According to Austin (1961), the egg is said to be "penetrated" or "undergoing fertilization" when in the early stage of fertilization, and a "fertilized egg" is one that has progressed at least to the metaphase of the first mitotic cleavage or is undergoing cleavage. Bearing these criteria in mind, but without severe restriction for description and discussion, this paper attempts to review the literature up to the present time and to examine the progress made in different species, with particular reference to the experience of the author.

Early Work on Rabbit Eggs

When a drop of epididymal sperm was added to the follicular eggs of rabbits suspended in follicular fluid together with uterine mucus, Schenk (1878) observed the dissolution of follicular cells adherent to the eggs. The breakup of the follicular granulosa cell mass by sperm suspensions has been confirmed subsequently by many workers (Yamane, 1930, 1935; Pincus, 1930, 1936) and probably led to the discovery of the presence of hyaluronidase in sperm (Fekete and Duran-Reynals, 1943; McClean and Rowlands, 1942). Schenk's use of uterine mucus or an excised piece of uterus is of interest, for this was a forerunner to the study of Smith (1951), who used scrapings from the Fallopian tubes in her *in vitro* preparation. Later work by Brackett and Williams (1968) demonstrated that the presence of uterine fluid could be also beneficial for accomplishment of fertilization *in vitro*.

Yamane (1930, 1935) working on follicular and tubal eggs of rabbits, reported the proteolytic action of mammalian spermatozoa and its bearing upon the second maturation division of eggs. He also claimed the possibility of fertilization *in vitro*, but the presence of

[1] Research Career Awardee of NICHD, PHS (K6 HD-18,334).

intact sperm heads in a distorted section of an egg (Yamane, 1935) is hardly convincing.

Pincus (1930) reported that when tubal rabbit eggs obtained from does previously mated to vasectomized bucks were incubated with sperm, a high proportion of eggs cleaved, but there was no significant difference in the proportion of cleaved eggs between the experimental (60%) and untreated (65%) control eggs. Although he claimed to have observed penetration of a spermatozoon into the vitellus in two eggs, according to Smith (1951), "it is unlikely that Pincus could have seen the passage of the spermatozoon through the corona radiata and the zona pellucida or into the egg." It should be mentioned here that in his original report Pincus (1930) did not claim to have achieved fertilization *in vitro*, but he (1936) did assume that the presence of two polar bodies was an adequate criterion of fertilization *in vitro*. It is now known that the division of the first polar body is quite common and that the chromatin of the second polar body after being stained is usually quite different from that of the first polar body (Chang, 1957). For this reason, it should be kept in mind that a fragment of the vitellus or the division of the first polar body can be quite easily mistaken for the second polar body. Pincus and Enzmann (1934) obtained offspring by transplantation of eggs assumed to have been fertilized *in vitro* into the tubes of a recipient rabbit. In this experiment they mixed freshly shed rabbit eggs with sperm *in vitro* for ½ hr. and then washed off the adherent sperm. As we know, washing newly shed eggs free of sperm is not an easy task; thus the possibility of fertilization by adherent sperm in the Fallopian tube in these experiments cannot be excluded.

In vitro fertilization of rabbit eggs by sperm of rabbit or rat was reported by Krasovskaja (1935). Since in this study rabbit eggs were recovered 17 hr. after copulation with vasectomized males when rabbit eggs are at the end of their fertilizable life (Hammond, 1934; Chang, 1952a), it is doubtful whether these eggs were capable of fertilization. It is known that spontaneous activation of eggs occurs at the time of or soon after the loss of their fertilizability in many species (Yanagimachi and Chang, 1961; Chang and Yanagimachi, 1963; Marston and Chang, 1964). Although rabbit eggs are more stable in this respect, it is possible that the apparent emission of the second polar body, the formation of pro-

nuclei or cleavage of the eggs described in this paper were the result of parthenogenetic activation rather than fertilization particularly as all manipulation of eggs was done at room temperature.

Moricard (1950, 1953, 1954, 1955) has claimed successful fertilization of rabbit eggs *in vitro*. He ligated the Fallopian tubes of virgin rabbits after induced ovulation and injected a small amount of freshly collected semen into the tube. The tube was then removed and incubated *in vitro* under vaseline oil for 7½ hr. Intact sperm heads were seen in histological sections of the zona pellucida and in the vitellus, but a second polar body and pronucleus were not observed. In the opinion of Smith (1951), "Moricard has achieved the first stage of fertilization, and he attributes this success to the relatively anaerobic conditions." It has been the experience of the present author that a mass of cellular debris generally appeared in the Fallopian tubes following their *in vitro* incubation with semen in the absence of antibiotics. Moreover, the enlargement of the fertilizing sperm head in the vitellus occurs very rapidly, and its transformation into the male pronucleus occurs only a few hours after penetration (Chang and Hunt, 1962). If the eggs photographed by Moricard were really penetrated, one would hardly have expected a distinctive intact sperm head in the vitellus. As we know, sperm heads can easily be transferred from one part of a histological section to another, either in the cutting of the sections or during the staining and mounting procedures. Thus the presence of an intact sperm head in the vitellus of a sectioned egg is not a convincing evidence for sperm penetration. In addition, Moricard (1950) reported the penetration of a spermatozoon into the ooplasm of five out of 21 eggs (24%) *in vitro* under relatively anaerobic conditions. Later he (1954) stated that about 30% of rabbit tubal eggs were fertilized by sperm recovered from the female tract. Since there is no great difference between these two results, it is not clear whether such fertilization was due to anaerobic conditions or to employment of uterine (capacitated) sperm.

Smith (1951) reported that in the presence of Fallopian tube mucosa, 11 of 35 rabbit eggs were penetrated under a coverslip-sealed preparation. The presence of a sperm head within the vitellus, the formation of a pronucleus and the cleavage of one egg after further culture were taken as evidences for sperm penetration. She admitted, however, that sperm penetration was not observed owing to the density of the surrounding corona radiata, and that cleavage might possibly have been parthenogenetic.

Venge (1953) reported fertilization of rabbit eggs in a glass tube under "partial anaerobic conditions". Although two litters were produced when these eggs were transferred into recipient rabbits, he concluded that the development was due to chance and not to controlled process.

Later Work on Rabbit Eggs Using Capacitated Sperm

The evidences that ejaculated or epididymal rabbit sperm have to undergo some kind of physiological change within the female tract before they are capable of passing through the zona pellucida (capacitation) (Austin, 1951, 1952; Chang, 1951, 1955a) have been of critical importance for the subsequent success of fertilization in vitro. Thibault and his associates (Dauzier et al.. 1954; Thibault et al., 1954; Dauzier and Thibault, 1956) reported successful fertilization of rabbit eggs in vitro by incubation of eggs with sperm recovered from the uterus (capacitated sperm). Their evidence for fertilization was, however, still based on histological examination of eggs. The validity and reliability of all the supposedly successful in vitro fertilization experiments have been questioned (Smith, 1951; Austin, 1951; Chang, 1957) because of the ambiguity of cytological criteria as evidence of fertilization. In 1957 the possibility of fertilization of mammalian eggs in vitro was still regarded as sub judice (Austin and Bishop, 1957). It was felt that unless living young could be obtained after transplanting such fertilized eggs into recipient rabbits, successful fertilization in vitro could not be held to be proven, since such eggs may be abnormally fertilized or may not be fertilized at all. Finally Chang (1959) obtained living young, genetically resembling their parents following the transplantation of rabbit eggs fertilized in vitro by incubation of newly ovulated eggs with capacitated sperm in a small Carrel flask for 4 hr. Since these eggs were also subcultured for another 18 hr. in 50% rabbit serum before their transfer into foster mothers, it was stated by Zuckerman (1959) that the evidence for fertilization of mammalian eggs in vitro was for the first time incontestable. This was confirmed later by Thibault and Dauzier (1961) and Bedford and Chang (1962).

According to Dauzier and Thibault (1961), for successful fertilization in vitro, the quality of sperm used is not so important as the condition of eggs at recovery or during manipulation. This is contradictory to our experience as we found that the quality of sperm was of importance (Bedford and Chang, 1962). Thibault and Dauzier (1960) have also reported that washing of eggs for a few hours prior to fertilization resulted in an overall increase in the fertilization rate. These observations have not been confirmed by Bedford and Chang (1962). There was, however certain theoretical interest in connection with their notion that the fertilizing power of sperm is inhibited by "fertilisine-like substances" released from the freshly ovulated egg which can be washed off. Furthermore, Thibault and Dauzier (1961) reported an "antifertilisine substance" produced in the female tract, which is very sensitive to the lack of oxygen, neutralizes the "fertilisine-like substance" of eggs and leaves the way clear for the sperm to stick to and penetrate the zona pellucida. Sperm-activating substances emanating from eggs have been well demonstrated in several marine species (Lillie, 1923), but the possibility of their presence in mammals should, for the present, be regarded with caution.

In vitro fertilization of rabbit eggs in tubal fluid was reported by Suzuki and Mastroianni (1965). Essentially following the procedures of Chang (1959), they incubated freshly ovulated eggs with capacitated sperm in tubal fluid on a depressed slide for 4 hr. and then subcultured these eggs in 10% serum for another 18 to 20 hr. Examined under a phase microscope, 31% of these eggs were considered to be definitely fertilized when ordinary mineral oil was used to cover the preparation. When mineral oil equilibrated with 5% carbon dioxide was used, as many as 64% of the eggs were fertilized. Thus, equilibration of the oil seal with carbon dioxide apparently improves the chance for successful fertilization of rabbit eggs in this in vitro system. Whether or not tubal fluid plays a beneficial role is still not clear, since no other fluid was used as a control in their study. It should be mentioned here that in one of their photographs a thin layer of mucin coat can be seen. According to our experience, corona radiata cells were usually still attached to the eggs 7 hr. after insemination in vitro and no mucin coat which arises in the tube can ever be seen on the zona pellucida of any eggs, even though they may have cleaved twice. It appears that they have succeeded in fertilizing rabbit eggs *in vitro* because 22% of these fertilized eggs could develop into 16-celled eggs when cultured further for 2 to 3 days (Suzuki, 1968).

In vitro fertilization of rabbit eggs was also reported by Brackett and Williams (1965) using the general procedures of Chang (1959). They reported that the proportion of eggs fertilized was higher (73%) when tubal eggs were incubated with capacitated sperm in the presence of fresh uterine fluid rather than stored tubal or uterine fluid (30 to 32%). Their later experiment (Brackett and

pellucida of newly ovulated rabbit eggs to swell and to become soft. The real importance of uterine fluid in connection with the sperm penetration during fertilization has yet to be examined.

The Fertilization Rate of Rabbit Eggs in Vitro

Concerning the fertilization rate of rabbit eggs *in vitro*, the percentages of eggs fertilized as reported by various workers in different laboratories are presented in table 1. It should be pointed out here that Dauzier *et al.* (1954)

TABLE 1. *IN VITRO* FERTILIZATION OF RABBIT EGGS BY CAPACITATED SPERM

Total no. of eggs used	No. of eggs fertilized + %	Special technique used	Investigators
209	52 (25%)	Locke's solution in glass tube with paraffin oil	Dauzier *et al.*, 1954
77	36 (47%) (41 activated, 53%)	Locke's solution in glass tube with paraffin oil	Thibault *et al.*, 1954
1587	217 (14%)	Locke's solution in glass tube with paraffin oil	Dauzier and Thibault, 1959
922	121 (13%)	Locke's solution in glass tube with paraffin oil	Thibault and Dauzier, 1960
532	353 (66%)	Eggs washed to remove "fertilisine"	Thibault and Dauzier, 1961
266	55 (21%)	With sperm for 4 hr., subculture in 50% for 18 hr.	Chang, 1959
74	42 (57%)	10% serum in acidic saline	Chang, 1959
158	90 (57%)	10% serum in acidic saline	Bedford and Chang, 1962
54	41 (76%)	Addition of glutathione	
124	79 (64%)	In tubal fluid on slide covered with oil equilibrated with CO_2	Suzuki and Mastroianni, 1965
73	53 (73%)	With fresh uterine fluid	Brackett and Williams, 1965

Williams, 1968) has shown that when sperm recovered from the uterus were washed free of uterine fluid, only 20% of the eggs were fertilized and these fertilized eggs were only able to cleave as far as two cells instead of four cells usually seen after further incubation. It appears that uterine fluid may have some beneficial effect for sperm penetration *in vitro*, but it has not been determined whether or not fresh tubal fluid is better than fresh uterine fluid. According to the experiences of the author, uterine fluid or uterine washing has the ability to cause the zona

in their first paper reported a fertilization rate of 25%. In the same year, probably due to their over-eagerness, Thibault *et al.* (1954) reported nearly 100% fertilization. Although only 13 to 14% fertilization was reported later by them (Dauzier and Thibault, 1959; Thibault and Dauzier, 1960), a 66% fertilization rate was obtained by washing off the "fertilisine" from eggs (Thibault and Dauzier, 1961). In our experiment (Chang, 1959; Bedford and Chang, 1962), a 21% fertilization rate was obtained when Krebs-Ringer bicarbonate solution was used but 57% when

10% serum in acidic saline was used. In the presence of glutathione, however, 76% of the eggs were fertilized (Bedford and Chang, 1962).

Suzuki and Mastroianni (1965) obtained a fertilization rate of 64% by covering the preparation with mineral oil equilibrated with 5% carbon dioxide while Brackett and Williams (1965) obtained a fertilization rate of 73% when fresh uterine fluid was used. Considering the fact that the best results obtained by several investigators in different laboratories ranged from 57 to 76%, one can hardly say whether the washing of eggs, using tubal, or uterine fluid really has any beneficial effect, especially if one considers the different ways of manipulation of sperm and eggs by these different investigators.

It is the experience of the present writer that. in one trial. all the eggs recovered from a rabbit can be fertilized, whereas only a few eggs can be fertilized in another experiment. Considering the fact that the rate of fertilization *in vivo* in the rabbit is never below 94% (Chang, 1952b; Adams, 1956), the lower rate of fertilization *in vitro* and the uncertainty of the results indicate that there is still a great deal to be learned concerning the fertilization *in vitro* of rabbit eggs.

Hamster and Other Mammalian Eggs

Despite the common use of rodents in the laboratory, only a few published studies have been directed toward fertilization *in vitro* of rodent eggs. Schenk (1878) first reported the extrusion of a polar body and subsequent cleavage of guinea pig eggs when epididymal sperm were added to the eggs *in vitro*. Onanoff (1893) recovered guinea pig eggs from the uterus and mixed them with sperm *in vitro* to observe their development, either in culture or in the abdominal cavity. We know now that the eggs have lost their fertilizability long before they reach the uterus.

Although successful fertilization of rat eggs *in vitro* has been attributed to Long (1912), his original paper reveals that he noted only dissolution of the follicular cell mass and emission of a polar body. Since fragmentation of eggs *in vitro* is a very common occurrence, his result appears questionable. As for the attempt to fertilize eggs of domestic species *in vitro*, Thibault and Dauzier (1961) have obtained three out of 51 sheep eggs and one out of 56 pig eggs fertilized *in vitro* after exposure to sperm recovered from the uterus.

Successful fertilization of golden hamster eggs, however, was reported recently by Yanagimachi and Chang (1963, 1964). They obtained eggs in the cumulus clot together with a small drop of tubal fluid under paraffin oil. These eggs were then incubated at 36–38° C. for 7 to 10 hr. with a small amount of sperm collected either from the uterus of mated females or directly from the epididymis. The presence of an enlarged sperm head or male pronucleus and of a sperm tail within or around the vitellus were taken as evidence of early fertilization. The fertilization rate was always significantly higher when sperm recovered from the uterus of females 4 to 5 hr. after mating (60%) were used rather than epididymal sperm (20 to 40%). The low fertilization rate following insemination with epididymal sperm was attributed to late penetration of eggs. Polyspermy, though very rare in the hamster (Austin, 1956), occurred commonly and the occurrence of supplementary sperm in the perivitelline space was also frequent in both fertilized and unfertilized eggs. Since about 45% of eggs were capable of dividing only once following subsequent culture, it appeared that the eggs were fertilized but were unable to sustain further cleavage under such experimental conditions. Further study of fertilization of hamster eggs *in vivo* and *in vitro* revealed that sperm penetration either *in vivo* or *in vitro* was earlier and faster in eggs exposed to sperm recovered from uterus rather than from the epididymis (Yanagimachi, 1966). In this latter study the whole process of sperm penetration *in vitro* was described and the time required for the sperm head to traverse the zona pellucida and the perivitelline space was determined to be 3 to 4 min. and 1 to 2 sec., respectively. This is probably the first reliable and authentic description of the sperm penetration of a mammalian egg.

The procedure for fertilization of hamster eggs *in vitro* conducted by Yanagimachi and Chang (1964) was confirmed by Barros and Austin (1967) who obtained a fertilization rate of 47% with epididymal sperm. They reported further that the fertilization rate is higher (47 to 66%) in the presence of follicular fluid or tubal fluid than in its absence brought about by washing (4.6%). The importance of follicular or tubal factors for successful *in vitro* fertilization of hamster eggs is, therefore, clearly demonstrated. In this connection, one may recall that the author (Chang, 1957) commented that "it seems that there are still other factors involved beside the capacitation of spermatozoa in the female tract" for the successful fertilization *in vitro.* "The motility of Fallopian tube and some unknown enzyme systems present in the tube which interact with sperm and eggs may play a role in mammalian fertil'zation." After 10 yr., it is very gratifying that some workers have demonstrated the importance of some tubal factors for the fertilization of mammalian eggs. It now remains for some biochemists to analyze the specific reaction of these factors which apparently facilitate fertilization.

Human Eggs

Human ovarian eggs were cultured *in vitro* for 24 hr. to induce maturation, and then were cultured further for 45 hr. in the presence of human sperm by Rock and Menkin (1944) and Menkin and Rock (1948). Altogether four of 138 eggs thus manipulated cleaved into two to three cells, whether or not these four eggs were really fertilized is still uncertain in view of the probability of the occurrence of some parthenogenetic cleavage during culture. Moreover, Rock and Menkin (1944) described that "at the end of incubation period, the more normal of two specimens consisted of three well-defined, round, regular blastomeres, each of which contained a round, vesicular nucleus." In this later case, one would have expected one of the three blastomeres to be at the stage immediately before division, and thus showing some evidence of mitotic chromosomes instead of a vesicular nucleus. Shettles (1955) reported the development of a human egg into morula after the incubation of an ovarian egg with human sperm and tubal mucosa *in vitro.* He neither excluded the possibility of artificial activation of the egg in his procedure nor mentioned the probability of parthenogenetic cleavage in his paper. Judging from the published photograph, it seems more likely that the "blastomeres" were simply fragments within the zona pellucida rather than those of a healthy morula.

Edwards (1965) reported that 80% of human oocytes recovered from women in various stages of menstrual cycle could mature from the post-dictyate stages to the extrusion of the first polar body by culturing them for 36 to 43 hr. When human oocytes thus cultured for 36 to 40 hr. were exposed to human sperm treated in various fashions, Edwards *et al.* (1966) reported that four of 56 oocytes were possibly fertilized by washed sperm, one of 14 by sperm previously placed in the rabbit uterus, two of 20 by sperms in the presence of endosalpinx. Since their evidence for fertilization was the presence of pronuclei, sperm tail, or the second polar body, whether these eggs were really penetrated or artificially activated is still in question. As shown in their photographs, the presence of one or two pronuclei without the identification of a sperm tail in the vitellus and that of polar bodies is not convincing evidence of fertilization because of the possibility of spontaneous formation of pronuclei in the unfertilized eggs. What may be a spermatozoon in the perivitelline space of one of their photographs does indicate, however, the possibility of sperm penetration through the zona pellucida. In this connection, Chang (1955) has reported that when oocytes of rabbits were first cultured for 12 hr. in serum, nuclear maturation (formation of the first polar body) was observed in the majority of the ovarian oocytes. Although a high percentage of these eggs were fertilized when transferred into the oviducts of mated rabbits, only two of 42 of such fertilized eggs were able to develop into normal young. Thus the acquisition of fertilizability of eggs and the possibility of their future development depends on the physiological state of the cytoplasm of the egg as a whole, and nuclear maturation is not necessarily an exact indication of their potential fertilizability.

Summary

The first attempt to fertilize mammalian eggs *in vitro* was made about 90 yr. ago, and the serious investigation of this problem was carried out about 30 yr. ago. Owing to overeagerness, the incomplete conception of the criteria of fertilization, and the lack of confirmation of the results, the likelihood of fertilization *in vitro* was still not acceptable. But we have learned a great deal from these masters. Before the recognition of capacitation some part of fertilization *in vitro* may have been achieved by some workers, but this was accomplished with certainty in the rabbit only after the recognition of the necessity for capacitation of sperm, about 16 yr. ago. The application of mineral oil on the preparation and the introduction of tubal or uterine fluid in the preparation appear to be beneficial for the successful fertilization *in vitro.* The successful fertilization of hamster eggs *in vitro,* and its confirmation in this year, leads us to look forward to the successful fertilization *in vitro* in other species. This depends on the achievement of capacitation of sperm *in vitro*, proper preparation of chemical media for the manipulation of sperm or egg at any stage and the best experimental procedure and conditions. Although the practical application of these techniques is still far off, with the present knowledge at our disposal, we anticipate a further clarification of the physiological and biological mechanisms involved in mammalian fertilization, particularly the reaction between sperm and eggs, the mechanism of sperm capacitation, the mechanism of sperm penetration, the behavior of pronuclei, and the integration of paternal and maternal materials within the egg.

Literature Cited

Adams, C. E. 1956. A study of fertilization in the rabbit: The effect of post-coital ligation of the Fallopian tube or uterine horn. J. Endoc. 13:296.

Austin, C. R. 1951. Observations on the penetration of the sperm into the mammalian egg. Australian J. Sci. Res. Ser. B, 4:581.

Austin, C. R. 1952. The capacitation of mammalian sperm. Nature 170:326.

Austin, C. R. 1956. Ovulation, fertilization and early cleavage in the hamster (*Mesocricetus auratus*). J. R. micr. Soc. 75:141.

Austin, C. R. 1961. Fertilization of mammalian eggs in vitro. Inter. Rev. Cytology, 12:337.

Austin, C. R. and M. W. H. Bishop. 1957. Fertilization in mammals. Biol. Rev. 32:296.

Barros, C. and C. R. Austin. 1967. *In vitro* fertilization of golden hamster ova. Anat. Rec. 157:209.

Bedford, J. M. and M. C. Chang. 1962. Fertilization of rabbit ova *in vitro*. Nature 193:898.

Brackett, B. G. and W. L. Williams. 1965. *In vitro* fertilization of rabbit ova. J. Exp. Zool. 160:271.

Brackett, B. G. and W. L. Williams. 1968. Fertilization of rabbit ova in a defined medium. Fertil. and Steril. (In press.).

Chang, M. C. 1951. Fertilizing capacity of sperm deposited in the Fallopian tube. Nature 168:697.

Chang, M. C. 1952a. Fertilizability of rabbit ova and effects of temperature *in vitro* on their subsequent fertilization and activation *in vivo*. J. Exp. Zool. 121:351.

Chang, M. C. 1952b. An experimental analysis of female sterility in the rabbit. Fertil. and Steril. 3:251.

Chang, M. C. 1955. Development of fertilizing capacity of rabbit spermatozoa in the uterus. Nature 175:1036.

Chang, M. C. 1957. Some aspects of mammalian fertilization. *In* A. Tyler, C. B. Metz and R. C. von Borstel [ed.] The Beginnings of Embryonic Development. American Association for the Advancement of Science.

Chang, M. C. 1959. Fertilization of rabbit ova *in vitro*. Nature 184:466.

Chang, M. C. and D. M. Hunt. 1962. Morphological changes of sperm head in the cop'asm of mouse, rat, hamster and rabbit. Anat. Rec. 142:417.

Chang, M. C. and G. Pincus. 1951. Physiology of fertilization in mammals. Physiol. Rev. 31:1.

Chang, M. C. and R. Yanagimachi. 1963. Fertilization

of ferret ova by deposition of epididymal sperm into the ovarian capsule with special reference to the fertilizable life of ova and the capacitation of sperm. J. Exp. Zool. 154:175.

Dauzier, L. and C. Thibault. 1956. Recherches expérimentales sur la maturation des gamètes mâles chez les mammifères, par l'étude de la fécondation *in vitro* de l'oeuf de lapine. Third Inter. Congr. An. Reprod., Cambridge.

Dauzier, L. and C. Thibault. 1959. Données nouvelles sur la fécondation *in vitro* de l'oeuf de la lapine et de la brebis. C. R. Acad. Sci., Paris. 248:2655.

Dauzier, L. and C. Thibault. 1961. La fécondation *in vitro* de l'oeuf de lapine. Fourth Inter. Congr. An. Reprod. and Art. Ins. The Hague.

Dauzier, L., C. Thibault and S. Wintenberger. 1954. La fécondation *in vitro* de l'oeuf de la lapine. C. R. Acad. Sci., Paris. 238:844.

Edwards, R. G. 1965. Maturation *in vitro* of human ovarian oocytes. Lancet 2:926.

Edwards, R. G., R. P. Donahue, T. A. Baramki and H. W. Jones. 1966. Preliminary attempts to fertilize human oocytes matured *in vitro*. Am. J. Obstet. and Gyn. 96:192.

Fekete, E. and F. Duran-Reynals. 1943. Hyaluronidase in the fertilization of mammalian ova. Proc. Soc. Exp. Biol. and Med. 52:119.

Hammond, J. 1934. The fertilization of rabbit ova in relation to time. A method of controlling the litter size, the duration of pregnancy and the weight of the young at birth. J. Exp. Biol. 11:140.

Krasovskaja, O. V. 1935. Cytological study of the heterogenous fertilization of the egg of rabbit outside the organism. Acta Zool. 16:449.

Lillie, F. R. 1923. Problems of Fertilization. The University of Chicago Press. Chicago, Illinois.

Long, J. A. 1912. The living eggs of rats and mice with a description of apparatus for obtaining and observing them. Univ. Cal. Pub. Zool. 9:105.

Marston, J. H. and M. C. Chang. 1964. The fertilizable life of ova and their morphology following delayed insemination in mature and immature mice. J. Exp. Zool. 155:237.

McClean, D. and I. W. Rowlands. 1942. The role of hyaluronidase in fertilization. Nature 150:627.

Menkin, M. F. and J. Rock. 1948. *In vitro* fertilization and cleavage of human ovarian eggs. Am. J. Obstet. and Gyn. 55:440.

Moricard, R. 1950. Penetration of the spermatozoa *in vitro* into the mammalian ovum oxydo potential level. Nature 165:763.

Moricard, R. 1953. Research on the formation of the second polar body in the tube after entrance of the sperm into the oocyte. *In* G. E. W. Wolstenholme [ed.] Mammalian Germ Cells. Ciba Foundation Symposium.

Moricard, R. 1954. Observation of *in vitro* fertilization in the rabbit. Nature 173:1140.

Moricard, R. 1955. La fonction fertilisatrice des secretions uterotubaires (étude microcinematographique de la fécondation *in vitro* de l'ovocyte de lapine.) *In* La Fonction Tubaire et Ses Trobles. Masson et Cie. Paris.

Onanoff, J. 1893. Recherches sur la fécondation et la gestation des mammifères. C. R. Soc. Biol., Paris. 45:719.

Pincus, G. 1930. Observations on the living eggs of the rabbit. Proc. Roy. Soc. B, 107:132.

Pincus, G. 1936. The Eggs of Mamma's. Exp. Biol. Monographs. Macmillan Co., New York.

Pincus, G. and E. V. Enzmann. 1934. Can mammalian

eggs undergo hormonal development *in vitro?* Proc. Nat. Acad. Sci. Wash. 20:121.

Rock, J. and M. F. Menkin. 1944. *In vitro* fertilization and cleavage of human ovarian eggs. Science 100:105.

Schenk, S. L. 1878. Das Säugethierei künstlich befruchtet ausserhalb des Mutterthieres. Mitth. Embryol. Inst. K. K. Univ. Wien. 1:107.

Smith, A. U. 1951. Fertilization *in vitro* of the mammalian egg. Biochem. Soc. Symp. no. 7.

Shettles, L. B. 1955. A morula stage of human ovum developed *in vitro.* Fertil. and Steril. 6:287.

Suzuki, S. 1968. *In vitro* cultivation of rabbit ova following *in vitro* fertilization in tubal fluid. Cytologica. (In press.).

Suzuki, S. and L. Mastroianni. 1965. *In vitro* fertilization of rabbit ova in tubal fluid. Am. J. Obstet. and Gyn. 93:465.

Thibault, C. and L. Dauzier. 1960. "Fertilisines" et fécondation *in vitro* de l'oeuf de lapine. C. R. Acad. Sci., Paris. 250:1358.

Thibault, C. and L. Dauzier. 1961. Analyse des conditions de la fécondation *in vitro* de l'oeuf de la lapine. Ann. Biol. An. Biochem. Biophys. 1:277.

Thibault, C., L. Dauzier, and S. Wintenberger. 1954. Etude cytologique de la fécondation *in vitro* de l'oeuf de la lapine. C. R. Soc. Biol., Paris. 148:789.

Venge, O. 1953. Experiments on fertilization of rabbit ova *in vitro* with subsequent transfer to alien does. *In* G. E. W. Wolstenholme [ed.] Mammalian Germ Cells. Ciba Foundation Symposium.

Yamane, J. 1930. The proteolytic action of mammalian spermatozoa and its bearing upon the second maturation division of ova. Cytologica 1:394.

Yamane, J. 1935. Kausal-analytische Studien über die Befruchtung des Kanincheneies. I. Die Dispersion der Follikelzellen und die Ablösung der Zellen der Corona radiata des Eies durch Spermatozoen. Cytologica 6:233.

Yanagimachi, R. 1966. Time and process of sperm penetration into hamster ova *in vivo* and *in vitro.* J. Reprod. Fertil. 11:359.

Yanagimachi, R. and M. C. Chang. 1961. Fertilizable life of golden hamster ova and their morphological changes at the time of losing fertilizability. J. Exp. Zool. 148:185.

Yanagimachi, R. and M. C. Chang. 1963. Fertilization of hamster eggs *in vitro.* Nature 200:281.

Yanagimachi, R. and M. C. Chang. 1964. *In vitro* fertilization of golden hamster ova. J. Exp. Zool. 156:361.

Zuckerman, S. 1959. Mechanisms involved in conception. Science 130:1260.

In Vitro Fertilization of Ovulated Rabbit Ova Recovered from the Ovary[1, 2]

H. M. SEITZ, JR.[3], BENJAMIN G. BRACKETT,
AND LUIGI MASTROIANNI, JR.

In 1951 Austin and Chang independently demonstrated the necessity for rabbit spermatozoa to undergo a form of conditioning within the female reproductive tract before acquiring the capacity to fertilize. The importance of this capacitation phenomenon in the *in vitro* fertilization of rabbit ova is well known. The possibility that the ovum itself undergoes some modification under the in-

fluence of the female reproductive tract as a prerequisite to fertilization has been suggested. In all previous work on the *in vitro* fertilization of rabbit ova using capacitated spermatozoa, the ova were recovered by flushing the oviducts, or follicular ova treated with tubal fluid were used (Brackett, 1969b). The purpose of this investigation was to evaluate the fertilizability of the ovulated rabbit ovum prior to exposure to any mechanical or biochemical influence of the oviduct.

[1] Presented at the First Annual Meeting of the Society for the Study of Reproduction, Nashville, Tennessee.

[2] Supported by Public Health Service Grants HD00130 and HD01810 and a grant from the Ford Foundation.

[3] United States Public Health Service Trainee under Public Health Service Grant HD00130.

METHODS AND MATERIALS

Mature New Zealand white rabbits weighing 3–5 kg were used. All rabbits were isolated for a minimum of 21 days to exclude the possibility of pseudopregnancy. Initial experiments were carried out to establish the expected interval between HCG injection and ovulation in does with and without prior treatment with PMSG. Direct observations of ovulation were made beginning just prior to the expected time of the initial ovulation. A Zeiss dissecting microscope was used by focusing through a 37C saline peritoneal bath.

Ovum donors were superovulated with 150 IU of PMS (Gestyl, Organon) given intramuscularly followed by 75 IU of HCG (APL, Ayerst) given intravenously 72–96 hr later. Nine and one-half hours after HCG injection the abdominal cavity of each ovum donor was opened. Intravenous pentobarbital was the mode of anesthesia used. Both fimbriae, including a portion of each ampulla, were resected (Fig. 1). The abdominal wall was then closed temporarily with Allis clamps and the animal was allowed to ovulate.

Eleven and one-half hr post-HCG injection, the ovaries were removed and placed immediately in normal saline at 37C (Fig. 2A). The ova were dissected from their ovulation sites in a 37C room. Cumulus masses containing the ova adhered to their stigmas, as was previously observed (Clewe, 1961).

Ova were dissected from the ovary with small probes in a saline bath under a dissecting microscope. Care was taken to avoid mechanical rupture of adjacent follicles. As each ovum was removed, it was transferred to a collecting dish to await insemination (Fig. 2B). Ovum recovery consumed approximately 40 min. Capacitated spermatozoa were then obtained by flushing the uterine horns of a rabbit doe (capacitator) mated 12 hr previously to bucks of proven fertility.

The defined synthetic medium of Brackett and Williams (1968) with 20% heat-inactivated rabbit serum added was used in the ovum collecting dish and for recovery of capacitated spermatozoa. The rabbit serum was heated at 55–60C for 20 min, and then refrigerated for periods not exceeding 2 weeks before use. The sperm suspension (4 ml) was placed in a sealable tissue culture dish (12 × 30 mm size, Bellco Glass, Inc., Vineland, New Jersey) under a layer of paraffin oil which was previously equilibrated with 5% CO_2-in-air atmosphere. Ova were transferred to the sperm suspension and the tissue-culture dish containing the gametes was wrapped in foil to avoid light and incubated at 37–38C in a 5% CO_2-in-air atmosphere. Under these conditions, when ova were

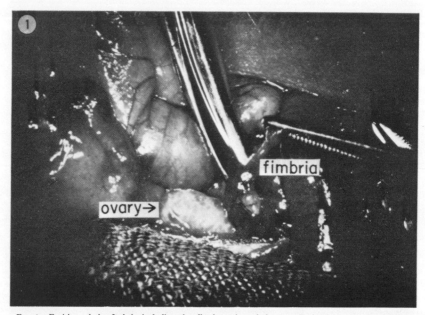

FIG. 1. Excision of the fimbria including the distal portion of the ampulla in the ovum donor prior to ovulation; ×10.

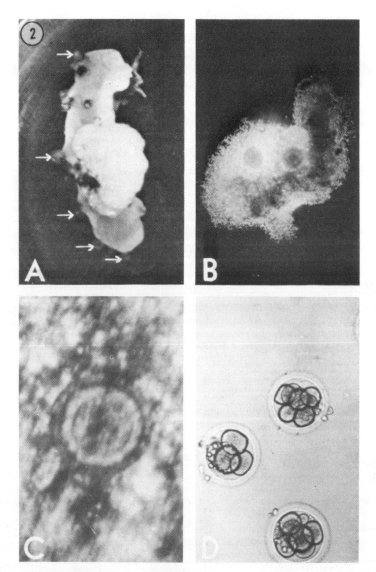

Fig. 2. A. Resected postovulatory rabbit ovary. Fimbria was removed proir to ovulation. Arrows indicate cumulus masses containing ova; ×15. B. Ova *in cumulus* after removal from ovulation sites on the ovary; ×50. C. Ovum as it appears 5 hr after insemination with capacitated spermatozoa. Note dispersal of cumulus cells; ×150. D. Representative cleaved ova 24 hr following insemination *in vitro*; ×100.

incubated with adequate numbers of capacitated spermatozoa, the cumulus dispersed within 5 hr (Fig. 2C).

During the initial phase of this investigation, 70 ova were examined for evidence of cleavage at various intervals after insemination. The remainder of the ova studied were examined 24-36 hr postinsemination (Fig. 2D). Ova which were not exposed to spermatozoa but subjected to the same experimental environment served as controls.

The criteria used for fertilization was normal zygote cleavage, or the birth of live young following the transfer of *in vitro* fertilized ova into recipient does, as previously reported by Chang (1959), Thibault, and Dauzier (1961) and Brackett (1969a).

RESULTS

The ovaries of 26 rabbits were studied by direct observation to determine the average time interval between intravenous injection of 75 IU of HCG and first ovulation. In 13 rabbits not treated previously with PMSG, the mean interval was found to be 10 hr and 35 min. In 13 animals receiving 150 IU of PMSG intramuscularly 72–96 hr prior to the HCG injection, the mean interval between HCG injection and initial ovulation was 10 hr and 7 min. The majority of follicles destined to ovulate did so within 11 hr and 30 min in both groups.

A total of 183 ova recovered directly from the surface of the ovary following ovulation were studied in this investigation. The first 70 ova were examined for cleavage at various time intervals following *in vitro* insemination (Table 1). Of those ova examined between 19 and 23 hr the majority were found to be

in the 2-cell stage. If examination was done between 24 and 30 hr, nearly 100% of the ova that cleaved were in the 4-cell stage. Thirty-two to 36 hr were required to obtain 8-cell ova. Seventy-three ova were checked for cleavage 24–26 hr postinsemination. Normal cleavage was observed in 117 of 143 ova incubated with capacitated spermatozoa. The *in vitro* rate of fertilization was, therefore, 81% (Table 2). None of 40 control ova, in four separate experiments, cleaved in the absence of spermatozoa.

Fertilization was confirmed in this experiment by the birth of one genetically dissimilar live young following the transfer of an *in vitro* fertilized ovum into a recipient doe. Of the two black checker rabbits used as recipients, the first showed two apparently normal implantations and a third undergoing regression 7 days after 3 *in vitro* fertilized ova were placed into her fallopian tubes. None of these implantations proceeded to term. The second recipient received three 4-cell ova and was not subjected to laparotomy during gestation.

TABLE 1

In Vitro DEVELOPMENT OF OVULATED OVA RECOVERED FROM THE OVARIAN SURFACE AND FERTILIZED *In Vitro*

Time following *in vitro* insemination of ova (hr)	Stage of ovum development			
	Not cleaved	2-Cell	4-Cell	8-Cell
19–23	2	6	2	0
25–30	11	2	25	0
36–38	4	4	2	12

TABLE 2

In Vitro FERTILIZATION OF OVULATED RABBIT OVA RECOVERED FROM THE OVARY

Experiment no.	Ova cleaved/ova recovered	% Normal cleavage[a]
7–1	4/5	80
7–2	6/9	66
7–3	8/8	100
7–4	5/8	62
7–5	4/5	80
7–6	7/9	77
7–7	6/9	66
7–8	4/5	80
7–9	9/12	75
7–10	15/19	79
7–11	16/17	94
7–12	8/8	100
7–13	7/9	77
7–14	3/4	75
7–15	5/6	83
7–16	10/10	100
Total	117/143	81

[a] Two- to eight-cell stage.

70

Twenty-nine days following ovum transfer, a white living offspring was born.

DISCUSSION

Direct observations of the ovulation process in this study agree with the investigation by Harper (1963) in which no ovulation took place by 10 hr, 50% of the ovulations occurred between 10.5 and 10.75 hr, and ovulation was complete by 14 hr after injection of 24 to 50 IU of HCG (Pregnyl, Organon). An interesting finding in the present investigation was that the time interval between HCG injection and the first ovulation can be reduced by previous treatment of the ovum donor with PMSG.

Previous studies have shown that washed tubal rabbit ova can be fertilized by washed uterine spermatozoa (Brackett, 1969a). In the hamster secretions in the female reproductive tract can be dispensed with for fertilization (Barros and Austin, 1967). The present data indicate that freshly ovulated rabbit ova recovered from the ovarian surface are capable of undergoing fertilization *in vitro* without any direct contact of the ovum with the oviduct. Recent observations indicate that the rabbit oviduct can be completely dispensed with for fertilization under *in vitro* conditions (Seitz *et al.*, 1969). These studies suggest that the essential contributions of the oviduct can be provided by a simple medium and controlled *in vitro* conditions. The medium contained a high concentration of bicarbonate and 20% serum, providing constituents which are present in the tubal secretions (Holmdahl and Mastroianni, 1965; David *et al.*, 1969). These constituents may be important in the fertilization process itself. The medium also might contain material brought in with the spermatozoa from the capacitator's uterus.

Austin and Braden (1954) found rabbit ova to be penetrated *in vivo* by spermatozoa very soon after ovulation, whereas a delay of 2–4 hr between ovulation and sperm penetration was observed in normally mated rats. This suggested that the rat ovum might require a final stage of maturation after ovulation before sperm penetration could occur. As no delay was observed in the rabbit, they concluded that maturation of the rabbit ovum is complete at ovulation. The present data lend support to their conclusion concerning the rabbit ovum. Sperm penetration of tubal rabbit ova under similar *in vitro* conditions occurs within the first 3 hr after insemination (Brackett, 1969c). Thibault and Dauzier (1961) have reported more rapid sperm penetration of rabbit ova *in vitro* following a 25–157 min period of washing the ova to remove a postulated "fertilizin." The time of sperm penetration under present conditions will be of interest since the recovery and pooling of recently ovulated ovarian ova prior to insemination required a time comparable to that used by Thibault and Dauzier (1961) in the ovum-washing step of their procedure.

Early cleavages were retarded by conditions of these experiments. The authenticity of fertilization and the potential for subsequent development of experimental ova were documented by the birth of a living offspring. In more recent experiments under similar conditions the lag in appearance of the early cleavage stages has been eliminated by transferring the ova from the sperm suspension after an initial 5 hr incubation (Seitz *et al.*, 1969).

ACKNOWLEDGMENTS

The authors wish to thank Mrs. Eva Kelly for her technical assistance and Mrs. Pamela Sundheim for assisting in the preparation of the manuscript.

REFERENCES

AUSTIN, C. R. (1950). Fertilization of the rat egg. *Nature* **166**, 407.

AUSTIN, C. R. (1951). Observations of the penetration of the sperm into the mammalian egg. *Aust. J. Sci. Res.* **B4**, 581.

AUSTIN, C. R., AND BRADEN, A. W. H. (1954). Time relations and their significance in the ovulation and penetration of eggs in rats and rabbits. *Aust. J. Biol. Sci.* **7**, 179–194.

BARROS, C., AND AUSTIN, C. R. (1967). *In vitro* fertilization and the sperm acrosome reaction in the hamster. *J. Exp. Zool.* **166**, 317–323.

BRACKETT, B. G., AND WILLIAMS, W. L. (1968). Fertilization of rabbit ova in a defined medium. *Fert. Steril.* **19**, 144–155.

BRACKETT, B. G. (1969a). Effects of washing the gametes on fertilization in vitro. *Fert. Steril.* **20**, 127–142.

BRACKETT, B. G. (1969b). *In vitro* fertilization of mammalian ova. In Raspe, G. (Ed.) Advances in the Biosciences 4, Schering Symposium on Mechanisms Involved in Conception, Berlin, 1969. Pergamon Press and Vieweg, New York, 1969.

BRACKETT, B. G. (1969c). *In vitro* fertilization of rabbit ova: time sequence of events. *Fert. Steril.* **21**, in press.

CHANG, M. C. (1951). Fertilizing capacity of spermatozoa deposited in the fallopian tubes. *Nature* **168**, 697–698.

CHANG, M. C. (1959). Fertilization of rabbit ova in vitro. *Nature* **184**, 466–467.

CLEWE, T. H. (1961). The attachment of the cumulus oophorus to the follicle after ovulation in the absence of the fimbria in rabbits. *Andt. Rec.* **139**, 217.

DAVID, A., BRACKETT, B. G., GARCIA, C-R., AND MASTROIANNI, L. (1969). Composition of rabbit oviduct fluid in ligated segments of the fallopian tube. *J. Reprod. Fert.* **19**, 285–289.

HARPER, M. J. K. (1963). Ovulation in the rabbit: the time of follicular rupture and expulsion of the eggs, in relation to injection of luteinizing hormone. *J. Endocrinol.* **26**, 307–316.

HOLMDAHL, T., AND MASTROIANNI, L. (1965). Continuous collection of rabbit oviduct secretions at low temperatures. *Fert. Steril.* **16**, 587–595.

SEITZ, H. M., JR., ROCHA, G., BRACKETT, B. G., AND MASTROIANNI, L. (1969). Influence of the oviduct on sperm capacitation in the rabbit. *Fert. Steril.* **21**, in press.

THIBAULT, C. AND DAUZIER, L. (1961). Analyse des conditions de la fecondation in vitro de l'oeuf de la lapine. *Ann. Biol. Anim. Biochem. Biophys.* **1**, 277–294.

Inhibition of *in Vitro* Fertilization of Rabbit Ova
by Trypsin Inhibitors

RICHARD STAMBAUGH, BENJAMIN G. BRACKETT,
AND LUIGI MASTROIANNI

Previous reports from our laboratory (Stambaugh and Buckley, 1968, 1969) have demonstrated that a trypsin-like enzyme, localized in the acrosome, is the zona pellucida penetration enzyme of rabbit sperm. Hyaluronidase, a mucopolysaccharidase also found associated with this trypsin-like enzyme, may possibly supplement the dissolution process, since the zona pellucida is a mucoprotein and contains small amounts of mucopolysaccharide. However, the trypsin-like component appears to be the more important component, since dissolution of the zona by the acrosomal extract can be completely inhibited by trypsin inhibitors. Also, it has been known for some time that proteolytic enzymes are capable of dissolving the zona pellucida, but hyaluronidase has no visible effect on this structure. The experiments described here were carried out to evaluate the ability of specific inhibitors of the acrosomal trypsin-like enzyme to prevent sperm from penetrating the zona pellucida of the rabbit ovum, and thus prevent union of the gametes.

METHODS AND MATERIALS

In previous publications (Stambaugh and Buckley, 1968, 1969) the trypsin-like acrosomal enzyme was

identified and characterized by its substrate specificity, its pH optimum, its sensitivity to specific inhibitors purified from natural sources (Worthington Biochemical Corporation, Freehold, New Jersey), and its dissolution action on the zona pellucida. In our previous publication (Stambaugh and Buckley, 1969) we described the subcellular localization of the trypsin-like enzyme in the acrosome. Extracts of isolated acrosomes were prepared in these experiments by sonication in 0.5% deoxycholate for 5 min at 0 C. After centrifugation the supernates were used to measure the inhibitory activity of the trypsin inhibitors.

Before selecting the inhibitors to be used for these *in vitro* experiments, their purity was first determined by polyacrylamide gel electrophoresis at 5 C. Electrophoresis was carried out with an EC 470 vertical gel electrophoresis apparatus with an 8% polyacrylamide gel prepared in pH 9.0 Tris buffer at 400 V for 1 hr, similar to methods previously applied to sperm lactic dehydrogenase (Stambaugh and Buckley, 1967). At the end of this time the positions of the protein bands were determined by staining with 0.5% amido black in 7% acetic acid for 15 min, and then destained with repeated washings with 15% acetic acid. The results of the electrophoretic analysis demonstrated that ovomucoid trypsin inhibitor was a highly purified protein, while soybean trypsin inhibitor showed only a trace of impurity in the electrophoretic pattern. The lima bean trypsin inhibitor, on the other hand, revealed no less than five distinct protein bands on electrophoresis. By eluting the major bands from the ovomucoid and soybean patterns, it was confirmed that the major band was the trypsin

TABLE 1

Inhibition of Crystalline Trypsin and
Chymotrypsin, and the Acrosomal
Trypsin-Like Enzyme by Soybean,
Lima Bean, and Ovomucoid
Trypsin Inhibitors

Trypsin inhibitor	Crystalline trypsin (% of uninhibited rate)	Crystalline chymotrypsin (% of uninhibited rate)	Acrosomal enzyme (% of uninhibited rate)
Soybean			
0 mg/ml	100	100	100
0.25 mg/ml	0.3	33	2
0.50 mg/ml	0.5	16	2
1.0 mg/ml	0.4	7	2
Lima bean			
0 mg/ml	100	100	100
0.25 mg/ml	0.6	0.3	2
0.50 mg/ml	0.6	0.5	1.8
1.0 mg/ml	0.6	0.6	1.8
Ovomucoid			
0 mg/ml	100	100	100
0.25 mg/ml	1.2	15	62
0.50 mg/ml	0.9	8	53
1.0 mg/ml	0.9	5	38

inhibitor. Lima bean trypsin inhibitor also showed less specificity for trypsin that the soybean inhibitor (Table 1). The low percentage inhibition by the ovomucoid inhibitor might logically be associated with its large molecular weight and steric factors of the bound acrosomal trypsin. Due to the impurity of the lima bean inhibitor, only the soybean and ovomucoid trypsin inhibitors were used in these experiments.

In vitro fertilization was carried out using methods similar to those described by Brackett and Williams (1968). Spermatozoa were capacitated *in vivo* for 12–13½ hr in rabbits injected intravenously with 50 IU of human chorionic gonadotropin. Ovum donors were primed with 150 U of Gestyl[1] intramuscularly 72 hr before ova collection and then superovulated with 50 IU of human chorionic gonadotropin 12 hr

[1] Gestyl—Gonadotrophic hormone from the serum of pregnant mares; Organon, Inc., West Orange, New Jersey.

This work was supported by Ford Foundation Grant 65-58A and by United States Public Health Service Grant HD 01810-04A1.

The authors gratefully acknowledge the technical assistance of Miss Susan Arenschield and Mrs. Eva Kelly.

before ova collection. Ova were flushed from the oviducts 12 hr later into watch glasses under paraffin oil; ova from one side served as the controls while those from the other side were used for the inhibition experiments. Manipulations of the ova were carried out in a tissue culture room at 37–38 C. Capacitated spermatozoa were recovered in 6.0 ml of the defined medium for each capacitator and pooled. This pooled sperm suspension was divided equally into two sealable-type tissue culture dishes, one containing the appropriate amount of inhibitor and the other, without inhibitor, serving as the control. Paraffin oil was layered over each dish, and the ova from donors were transferred to 4.0 ml of the appropriate sperm suspension.

After 4½ hr the ova were transferred to 4.0 ml of synthetic acidic medium containing 10% heated rabbit serum, 50 U of penicillin G, and 0.25% glucose. Incubation was carried out in this medium at 37–38 C in a Petri dish without gassing for 20 hr more. At the end of this time the ova were transferred to a slide, pressed under a cover glass, and examined by phase contrast microscopy. Fertilization was evidenced by normal cleavage. When there was any doubt about fertilization, the ova were stained with 1% lacmoid and reexamined to determine if each blastomere contained chromatin.

RESULTS

The effects of the presence of soybean and ovomucoid trypsin inhibitors are shown in Table 2. Apparently, a concentration of 1.0 mg/ml of soybean trypsin inhibitor is necessary to achieve good inhibition of fertilization. This level is not surprising, since inhibition of the enzymic activity is not complete at these concentrations (Table 1), and since the enzyme probably exists in a highly concentrated form on the sperm acrosomal membrane. Steric factors, preventing free access of the inhibitor to the enzyme, must also be considered as a possible cause for incomplete inhibition in these experiments. Throughout these experiments, no abnormalities of the unfertilized ova or presence of sperm in the zona pellucida or perivitelline space were discernible.

Figure 1 summarizes graphically the comparative effectiveness of the inhibitors on the isolated acrosomal enzyme with their effectiveness on *in vitro* fertilization. The results indicate that there is, indeed, a close correla-

TABLE 2

INHIBITION OF *in Vitro* FERTILIZATION OF RABBIT OVA BY TRYPSIN INHIBITORS

	Control (No inhibitor)		+ Inhibitor		
	Ova cleaved	Fert.	Ova cleaved	Fert.	Inhibition
Inhibitor	Ova recovered	(%)	Ova recovered	(%)	(%)
Soybean					
0.25 mg/ml	3/10	30	7/16	44	0
0.50 mg/ml	35/47	75	5/35	14	81
0.75 mg/ml	12/16	75	6/17	35	53
1.0 mg/ml	39/96	41	4/105	4	90
Ovomucoid					
1.0 mg/ml	40/53	75	34/71	48	36

tion between inhibition of the acrosomal trypsin-like enzyme and inhibition of *in vitro* fertilization, providing additional evidence that the trypsin-like enzyme of the acrosome is the essential enzyme for penetration of the zona pellucida of the rabbit ovum.

DISCUSSION

Srivastava, Adams, and Hartree (1965a, 1965b) have demonstrated a corona cell dispersing effect and sometimes a zona pellucida dissolution action of lipoglycoprotein preparations from rabbit sperm acrosomes. Since

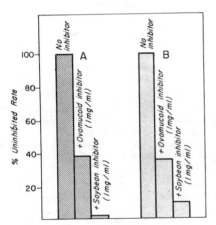

FIG. 1. Comparison of the percentage inhibition of the acrosomal trypsin-like activity (A) with the percentage inhibition of *in vitro* fertilization by ovomucoid and soybean trypsin inhibitors (B).

their extracts showed some proteolytic activity, they assumed that the zona dissolution may have been effected by these enzymes, although the proteolytic enzymes were not identified. Sperm extracts which disperse the corona radiata cells have also been reported by Zaneveld, McRorie, and Williams (1968).

The morphological aspects of sperm passage through the zona have been described extensively by Dickmann (1964, 1965), Dickmann and Dzuik (1964), Dzuik and Dickmann (1965), and Bedford (1968) in the rabbit, pig, and sheep; and by Austin (1951), and Austin and Bishop (1958) in the rat and other rodents. A great deal of similarity was observed between these species in that the sperm all followed a curved path through the zona. Austin (1963) and Bedford (1968) in electron microscopic studies on the rabbit found that the penetrating spermatozoon does not lose its entire acrosome, but instead retains the inner membrane around the anterior part of the sperm nucleus. According to the observation of Dzuik and Dickmann (1965), the factor in determining the penetration curve is the sperm penetration filament (SPF), which originates from the inner acrosomal membrane. Bedford (1967), on the other hand, could observe no evidence for a penetration filament on any one of 50 sperm in the process of traversing the zona pellucida of rabbit ova. Regardless of whether or not a penetration filament is formed from the inner acrosomal membrane, all of the available

75

evidence indicates that fusion and vesiculation of the outer acrosomal membrane with the plasma membrane, as observed by Barros, Bedford, Franklin, and Austin (1967), precede penetration of the zona pellucida by the spermatozoon.

Since the sperm do not all penetrate the zona in one direction, it would appear that the physiochemical makeup of the zona does not influence the sperm pathway. As the spermatozoon begins to penetrate the zona, an area of digestion is often seen in advance of the sperm head. One must conclude from these morphological observations that the curved penetration slit in the zona pellucida arises from degradative enzymes present in the sperm acrosome or on its inner membrane. Since the thickness of the slit made by the spermatozoon is quite narrow, one can also surmise that these degradative enzymes may be bound firmly to the sperm during their enzymic action. If they were released into solution, a much larger and less uniform penetration slit might be expected.

Previously, we described the identification and subcellular localization of a trypsin-like enzyme in the acrosomes of rabbit sperm, which effected rapid dissolution of the zona pellucida of rabbit ova (Stambaugh and Buckley, 1968, 1969). This enzyme occurred in combination with hyaluronidase as a complex molecule which sedimented in sucrose gradients in the region of proteins with molecular weights of approximately 59,000. Interestingly, Borders and Raftery (1968) recently reported the purification of testicular hyaluronidase as a complex glycoprotein molecule with a molecular weight of 61,000 as determined by gel filtration. Previous estimations of the molecular weights of testicular hyaluronidase have been in the region of 11,000 (Hogberg, 1954), indicating that Borders and Raftery (1968) may have isolated the same complex molecule from the developing sperm of the testes as we did from epididymal and ejaculated sperm. However, no assay for trypsin activity was carried out in their experiments.

The experiments described here provide additional evidence that the trypsin-like enzyme of the rabbit sperm acrosome is, indeed, essential for penetration of the zona pellucida. The relatively high concentrations of inhibitor needed to prevent fertilization are not disturbing, since these inhibitors must exist in a highly concentrated form on the inner acrosomal membrane or on the sperm penetration filament.

REFERENCES

AUSTIN, C. R. (1951). Observations on the penetration of the sperm into the mammalian egg. *Australian J. Sci. Res. (Ser. B)* **4**, 581–596.

AUSTIN, C. R. (1963). Acrosome loss from the rabbit spermatozoon in relation to entry into the egg. *J. Reprod. Fertility* **6**, 313–314.

AUSTIN, C. R. AND BISHOP, M. W. H. (1958). Role of the rodent acrosome and perforatorium in fertilization. *Proc. Roy. Soc. (London) (Ser. B)* **149**, 241–248.

BARROS, C., BEDFORD, M., FRANKLIN, L. E., AND AUSTIN, C. R. (1967). Membrane vesiculation as a feature of the mammalian acrosome reaction. *J. Cell Biol.* **39**, C1–C5.

BEDFORD, J. M. (1967). Experimental requirement for capacitation and observations of ultra-structural changes in rabbit spermatozoa during fertilization. *J. Reprod. Fertility (Supp.)* **2**, 35–48.

BEDFORD, J. M. (1968). Ultrastructural changes in the sperm head during fertilization in the rabbit. *Am. J. Anat.* **123**, 329–355.

BORDERS, C. L., JR., AND RAFTERY, M. A. (1968). Purification and partial characterization of testicular hyaluronidase. *J. Biol. Chem.* **243**, 3756–3762.

BRACKETT, G. B. AND WILLIAMS, W. L. (1968). Fertilization of rabbit ova in a defined medium. *Fertility Sterility* **19**, 144–155.

DICKMANN, Z. (1964). The passage of spermatozoa through and into the zona pellucida of the rabbit egg. *J. Exptl. Biol.* **41**, 177–182.

DICKMANN, Z. (1965). Sperm penetration into and through the zona pellucida of the mammalian egg. CIBA Found. *Symp. on Pre-implantation Stages of Pregnancy*, pp. 169–182.

DICKMANN, Z. AND DZUIK, P. J. (1964). Sperm penetration of the zona pellucida of the pig egg. *J. Exptl. Biol.* **41**, 603–608.

DZUIK, P. J. AND DICKMANN, Z. (1965). Sperm penetration through the zona pellucida of the sheep egg. *J. Exptl. Zool.* **158**, 237–239.

HOGBERG, B. (1954). The use of ion-exchange resin in the purification of hyaluronidase. *Acta Chem. Scand.* **8**, 1098.

SRIVASTAVA, P. N., ADAMS, C. E., AND HARTREE, E. T. (1965a). Enzymatic action of lipoglycoprotein preparations from sperm-acrosomes on rabbit ova. *Nature* **205**, 498.

SRIVASTAVA, P. N., ADAMS, C. E., AND HARTREE, E. T. (1965b). Enzymatic action of acrosomal preparations on the rabbit ovum *in vitro*. *J. Reprod. Fertility* **10**, 61–67.

STAMBAUGH, R. AND BUCKLEY, J. (1967). The enzymic and molecular nature of the lactic dehydrogenase subbands and X_4 isozyme. *J. Biol. Chem.* **242**, 4053–4059.

STAMBAUGH, R. AND BUCKLEY, J. (1968). Zona pellucida dissolution enzymes of the rabbit sperm head. *Science* **161**, 585–586.

STAMBAUGH, R. AND BUCKLEY, J. (1969). Identification and subcellular localization of the enzymes effecting penetration of the zona pellucida by rabbit spermatozoa, *J. Reprod. Fertility* **19**, 423–432.

ZANEVELD, L. J. D., McRORIE, R. A., AND WILLIAMS, W. L. (1968). A sperm enzyme that removes the corona radiata from ova and its inhibition by decapacitation factor. *Federation Proc.* **27**, 567.

77

FERTILIZATION OF CHINESE HAMSTER EGGS
IN VITRO

STELLA PICKWORTH AND M. C. CHANG

Fertilization of eggs *in vitro* has been described in three mammalian species—the rabbit (Dauzier, Thibault & Wintenberger, 1954; Chang, 1959; Suzuki & Mastroianni, 1965; Brackett & Williams, 1965), Syrian hamster (Yanagimachi & Chang, 1964; Barros & Austin, 1967) and laboratory mouse (Whittingham, 1968). Penetration by spermatozoa and pronucleus formation have also been observed in rat eggs, following dissolution of the zona pellucida by chymotrypsin (Toyoda & Chang, 1968).

In preliminary attempts to fertilize eggs of the Chinese hamster, *Cricetulus griseus, in vitro*, no success was achieved using fresh spermatozoa, but 10% of eggs (8 of 80) were penetrated by spermatozoa which had previously been incubated with Syrian hamster cumulus clot. This treatment was used in a larger study in August 1968, as described here.

Immature and maturing Chinese hamsters, 5 to 8 weeks old, were injected intraperitoneally with 5 i.u. PMSG (Equinex, Ayerst) followed 48 to 52 hr later by 10 i.u. HCG (A.P.L., Ayerst). Tubal eggs were recovered from females killed $15\frac{1}{2}$ to $16\frac{1}{2}$ hr after HCG and, from earlier studies, these were considered to be not more than 2 hr post-ovulation. Follicular eggs were obtained from females where ovulation had not begun or only a few follicles ruptured at this time, and from one female killed $14\frac{1}{2}$ hr after HCG. Syrian hamster cumulus clot was used for all pre-treatments of spermatozoa. It was obtained from superovulated mature females (Greenwald, 1962) killed on Day 4 of the cycle, $14\frac{1}{2}$ to $15\frac{1}{2}$ hr after injection of 10 i.u. HCG; about half the cumulus from one oviduct was used for each preparation.

Chinese hamster spermatozoa were stripped from the vas deferens into mineral oil and added to 1 ml of either Tyrode's solution or TC medium Ham F10 containing 1% bovine serum albumin. A drop of the suspension, 1 to 2 times the volume of the cumulus and containing approximately 4 to 6 million spermatozoa/ml, was then added to the Chinese hamster eggs or to Syrian hamster material for pre-incubation. Eggs for culture with the pre-treated spermatozoa were recovered from Chinese hamster females 2 to 3 hr later and added to the pre-incubation mixture. They were easily distinguished from the Syrian hamster eggs by their smaller size, as well as a different appearance of the cytoplasm, polar bodies and chromatin. All incubations were carried out at 37 to 38° C under mineral oil equilibrated with 5% CO_2 in air. Chinese hamster eggs were examined after $5\frac{1}{2}$ to 8 hr in contact with spermatozoa.

The highest number of penetrated eggs was observed after incubation of tubal eggs with pre-treated spermatozoa in F10+albumin (Table 1). Fertilizing spermatozoa were present on 45% of eggs in the ten successful cultures. Eggs undergoing normal fertilization had a second polar body, enlarged perivitelline space and two pronuclei. None of the eggs showed a sperm flagellum in the cytoplasm. Usually the anterior end of the sperm midpiece was attached to the vitelline membrane while the sperm tail and part of the midpiece lay outside the zona pellucida (Pl. 1, Fig. 1). Seven activated eggs, all from culture in Tyrode's solution, showed no trace of a male pronucleus or sperm structure. Fifteen other eggs, with no flagellum attached to them, contained what appeared to be both male and female pronuclei (Pl. 1, Fig. 2) and had probably been penetrated by spermatozoa. Incomplete entry of the fertilizing spermatozoon and absence of the sperm tail from cleaving eggs had been observed after fertilization *in vivo*, although in a smaller proportion of eggs (Pickworth, Yerganian & Chang, 1968).

Two or more 'subnuclei' replaced the normal female pronucleus in some of the activated eggs (Pl. 1, Fig. 3), suggesting that scattering of chromosomes had occurred. Fertilizing spermatozoa were present on sixteen of the twenty eggs showing this abnormality, and male pronuclear appearance was normal. Pronucleus formation was well advanced in most fertilized eggs. Enlarging sperm heads were found in six monospermic eggs, three of which contained large female pronuclei and therefore showed an abnormal sequence of development. One polyspermic egg was found after culture in Tyrode's solution, and thirteen (23% of activated eggs) in F10+albumin. All but one polyspermic egg came from cultures with pre-incubated spermatozoa.

No Syrian hamster eggs were penetrated by Chinese hamster spermatozoa, nor were spermatozoa adhering to the zona pellucida after incubation.

Syrian hamster cumulus was used for pre-treatment of spermatozoa in this study to conserve the more limited supply of Chinese hamsters for the main incubations. Excellent motility was observed with the Syrian hamster material. Incubation with tubal or follicular contents from other species has been shown to induce capacitation of Syrian hamster spermatozoa *in vitro*, resulting in more rapid penetration of eggs added to the culture after this period (Barros, 1968; Yanagimachi, 1969). In the Chinese hamster there is probably an interval of 2 hr or more between ovulation and sperm penetration *in vivo* (Pickworth *et al.*, 1968). No timing of sperm entry was attempted in the present series *in vitro*. However, it seems likely that important changes in the spermatozoa were initiated during pre-incubation, and the difference between results from fresh and pre-incubated spermatozoa may have arisen from a short fertilizable life of the eggs in culture.

Both fresh and pre-incubated spermatozoa showed good motility in culture with Chinese hamster tubal eggs. By contrast, the activity of spermatozoa with Chinese hamster follicular contents was severely reduced, and restricted to a narrow border zone around the preparation. The effect of follicular material from untreated mature females was not investigated.

This work supported by grants from U.S.P.H.S. and the Ford Foundation. The Chinese hamsters were kindly provided by Dr G. Yerganian, Children's Cancer Research Foundation, Boston.

REFERENCES

BARROS, C. (1968) *In vitro* capacitation of golden hamster spermatozoa with Fallopian tube fluid of the mouse and rat. *J. Reprod. Fert.* **17,** 203.

BARROS, C. & AUSTIN, C. R. (1967) *In vitro* fertilization and the sperm acrosome reaction in the hamster. *J. exp. Zool.* **166,** 317.

BRACKETT, B. G. & WILLIAMS, W. L. (1965) *In vitro* fertilization of rabbit ova. *J. exp. Zool.* **160,** 271.

CHANG, M. C. (1959) Fertilization of rabbit ova *in vitro*. *Nature, Lond.* **184,** 466.

DAUZIER, L., THIBAULT, C. & WINTENBERGER, S. (1954) La fécondation *in vitro* de l'oeuf de la lapine. *C. r. Acad. Sci., Paris,* **238,** 844.

GREENWALD, G. S. (1962) Analysis of superovulation in the adult hamster. *Endocrinology,* **71,** 378.

PICKWORTH, S., YERGANIAN, G. & CHANG, M. C. (1968) Fertilization and early development in the Chinese hamster, *Cricetulus griseus. Anat. Rec.* **162,** 197.

SUZUKI, S. & MASTROIANNI, L. (1965) In vitro fertilization of rabbit ova in tubal fluid. *Am. J. Obstet. Gynec.* **93,** 465.

TOYODA, Y. & CHANG, M. C. (1968) Sperm penetration of rat eggs *in vitro* after dissolution of zona pellucida by chymotrypsin. *Nature, Lond.* **220,** 589.

WHITTINGHAM, D. G. (1968) Fertilization of mouse eggs *in vitro*. *Nature, Lond.* **220,** 592.

YANAGIMACHI, R. (1969) *In vitro* capacitation of hamster spermatozoa by follicular fluid. *J. Reprod. Fert.* **18,** 275.

YANAGIMACHI, R. & CHANG, M. C. (1964) *In vitro* fertilization of golden hamster ova. *J. exp. Zool.* **156,** 361.

EXPLANATION OF PLATE 1

Phase contrast. Figs. 1 and 2: fresh specimens, compressed; × 268. Figs. 3 and 4: fixed, stained with lacmoid; × 201.

FIG. 1. Egg of normal penetrated appearance showing second polar body, male (left) and female (right) pronuclei; anterior end of sperm flagellum attached to the vitelline membrane.

FIG. 2. Egg showing second polar body and pronuclei comparable with Fig. 1; no sperm flagellum attached at the time of examination.

FIG. 3. Penetrated egg showing sperm midpiece and male pronucleus (a) but containing two small female pronuclei adjacent to the second polar body (b).

FIG. 4. Egg showing a partially enlarged sperm head (a), second polar body (a, upper right) and large female pronucleus (b).

PLATE 1

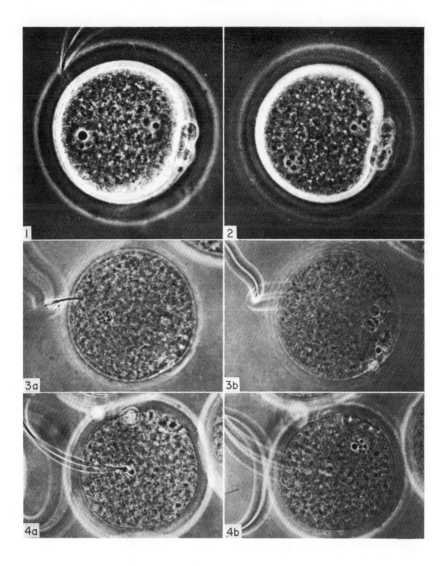

TABLE 1

FERTILIZATION OF CHINESE HAMSTER EGGS IN VITRO; EFFECT OF PRE-INCUBATION OF SPERMATOZOA

Medium	Source of eggs	Sperm. pre-inc. (hr)	No. of cultures		No. of eggs				
			Total	With penetrated eggs	Total	Activated*	Fertilizing sperm. present	Fertilized? no sperm. flagellum	No male component
F10 with 1% b.s.a.	Oviduct	—	9	1	97	6	6	—	—
	Oviduct	2 to 3	21	10	192	51	42 (22%)	9	—
	Follicles	2 to 3	3	—	25	—	—	—	—
Tyrode's solution	Oviduct	2 to 3	17	11	168	29	17 (10%)	6	6
	Follicles	2 to 3	10	—	71	1	—	—	1

* By spermatozoa or other stimulus.

82

FERTILIZATION OF MOUSE OVA *IN VITRO*

I. EFFECT OF SOME FACTORS ON FERTILIZATION

ANTONÍN PAVLOK

INTRODUCTION

Fertilization of mouse ova *in vitro* has so far been successful only in explanted ampullar parts of oviducts (Brinster & Biggers, 1965). The proportion of ova fertilized was comparatively small, although the development of fertilized mouse eggs in explanted oviducts (Biggers, Gwatkin & Brinster, 1962) has been shown to proceed without greater loss up to the blastocyst stage (Gwatkin, 1962).

The need for oocytes to spend some time in the oviduct before penetration can occur has not been proved yet, though it could be assumed from the communications of Thibault & Dauzier (1960, 1961). The time which spermatozoa spend in the female genital tract before fertilization seems important for their ability to penetrate the membranes of ova, especially in rabbits (Chang 1951, 1957; Austin, 1951, 1952). In hamsters this capacitation process appears to be considerably quicker or even unnecessary (Yanagimachi & Chang, 1964). The interval between copulation and penetration of ova is also short in mice (Braden & Austin, 1954; Krzanowska, 1966). None the less, in-vitro fertilization of mouse ova appears to need far more specific conditions than in hamsters.

The aim of this paper was to investigate the effect of some factors on the fertilization of mouse ova in explanted ampullar parts of oviducts, and to obtain a higher percentage of fertilized eggs by a suitable modification of the fertilizing conditions.

MATERIAL AND METHODS

One hundred and thirty-three female mice, 10 to 15 weeks old, of the inbred strain C57BL/10 Sc Sn, and F_1 and F_2 progeny of C57BL/10 Sc Sn females and A males were used for the experiments. For individual experiments, groups of females homogeneous in age and origin were chosen. Ovulation was induced by 6 to 8 i.u. PMSG (Bioveta) and 20 to 25 i.u. HCG (Praedyn—Spofa). The spermatozoa used for fertilization of ova *in vitro* were taken from F_1 progeny of C57BL/10 Sc Sn females and A males.

The medium for cultivation of oviducts was similar in its composition to the medium BGJb, used by Biggers *et al.* (1962) and Brinster & Biggers (1965). Medium TC 199 was supplemented with glucose, sodium lactate and $NaHCO_3$, as well as with other theoretically useful components, to be tested for their effect on fertility. The complete medium, pH 7·8 to 8·1, was composed of the following components:

TC 199 (Usol) (Isotonic solution)	50%
Earle's solution with 0·3% lactalbumin hydrolysate (Usol)	4%
Solution of $NaHCO_3$ (1·32%)	16%
Solution of glucose (6·2%)	7%
Solution of sodium lactate (1·74%)	3%
Tyrode's solution with 0·268% glycine	20%

This medium was made from previously prepared stock solutions, completed by 100 i.u. of penicillin and 50 i.u. of streptomycin/ml. When one of the components was to be tested, it was either completely omitted from the medium or included in minimal concentration.

The technique of organ culture on agar was described by Trowell (1959). The stock solution for agar sheet preparation was obtained by dissolving 2 g of agar in 100 ml of 0·7% NaCl. The sterile heated agar solution was poured in a 3-mm thick layer into a Petri dish, 6 cm in diameter, and left to cool. Two agar sheets were made from one Petri dish. When preparing Petri dishes for culture, two glass rods, about 3 mm thick and bent at a right angle, were placed at the bottom of the dish, with the function of agar sheet carriers. When the medium was poured into the dish, the agar sheet, occupying about 40% of the surface, was carefully placed on the glass rods and the dish was filled up to the upper edges of the sheet.

Superovulated females were killed 14 to 16 hr after the administration of HCG, except in the experiment in which the effect of pH on fertilization rate of ova was studied, when the females were killed 13 to 17 hr after the administration of HCG. Oviducts were removed aseptically with the ovaries and parts of uterine horns, and undamaged ampullar parts with about three spirals of the isthmal part were prepared under the stereomicroscope. When oviducts were shortened too much, cultivated ova were often expelled. Preliminary experiments showed that mass lysis of ova could be caused by injury to the wall of the ampullar part of the oviduct, especially the infundibulum. For insemination, oviducts were rinsed with cultivating medium and transferred to a previously prepared suspension of spermatozoa for a period of 9 to 10 min.

The suspension of uterine spermatozoa was obtained from the uteri of intact superovulated females 2 to 4 hr after copulation. Spermatozoa isolated 1 to 7 hr after copulation were used when evaluating the fertility of spermatozoa in relation to the period of their stay in the uterus. Uterine spermatozoa were diluted in 0·1 ml of medium in paraffin oil to a concentration of about 300 to 5000 spermatozoa/mm³.

After incubating in the suspension of spermatozoa, oviducts were transferred on to agar sheets and cultivated at 37·5° C and about 90% humidity, in an atmosphere of 5% CO_2 in oxygen or air. Oviducts were cultured on agar sheets for 18 to 22 hr, except for the experiment in which the effect of sodium lactate and glucose on fertilization rate and subsequent development of ova was studied (Table 3), when the time of cultivation was prolonged to 48 hr. After cultivation, the oviducts were flushed, and the ova examined by means of a fluorescent microscope (Austin & Bishop, 1959) and classified into fertilized and unfertilized. Ova with two or more pronuclei, ova in the process of syngamy and ova with two or more blastomeres were classified as fertilized. The second polar body was also observed in all ova considered as fertilized. The process of fragmentation of unfertilized ova was carefully studied in preliminary experiments, so that it would not be confused with cleavage.

To evaluate the influence of the tested factors, one oviduct of each female was used as experimental, the other as control. Statistical evaluation was carried out by means of the t-test, after angular transformation of results according to Fisher & Yates (1953). The effect of uneven numbers of ova in the experimental and control groups was allowed for by an appropriate correction.

RESULTS

In the first experiment, the effect of inactivated homologous serum on the fertilization of ova in explanted ampullar parts of oviducts was tested. Five to 10% of inactivated homologous serum (30 min at 56° C) was added to the medium intended for insemination and also to the culture medium. The same medium, but without serum, served as a control. The differences between the percentage of ova fertilized in the experimental and control media were not significant (Table 1).

The use of a higher concentration of glycine in the medium for the fertilization of ova in vitro was suggested by a communication from Gregoire, Gondskadi & Rakoff (1961), who found that glycine is the most widely distributed free amino acid of the oviducal secretion in rabbits. Our test medium contained glycine at a concentration of 56·1 mg%, the control 2·5 mg%. The higher concentration of free glycine did not influence the percentage of ova fertilized (Table 2).

The importance of sodium lactate as an energy source during fertilization and the initial stages of development of ova in explanted oviducts was tested at a concentration of 52·2 mg% which is approximately the same as the concentration of calcium lactate in the medium BGJb (55·5 mg%). The percentage

TABLE 1

FERTILIZATION RATE OF OVA IN MEDIUM WITH AND WITHOUT SERUM

Serum (%)	No. of oviducts	No. of ova		% ova fertilized	P
		Isolated	Fertilized		
5 to 10	14	190	103	54·2	> 0·10
0	14	186	92	49·5	

TABLE 2

FERTILIZATION RATE OF OVA IN MEDIUM CONTAINING DIFFERENT AMOUNTS OF GLYCINE

Glycine (mg%)	No. of oviducts	No. of ova		% ova fertilized	P
		Isolated	Fertilized		
56·1	12	198	113	57·6	> 0·10
2·5	12	179	99	55·3	

TABLE 3

EFFECT OF SODIUM LACTATE AND GLUCOSE ON FERTILIZATION RATE AND FURTHER DEVELOPMENT OF OVA

Medium	No. of oviducts	No. of ova		% ova fertilized	P	No. of ova 5 to 8 blastomere after 48 hr	% ova 5 to 8 blastomere
		Isolated	Fertilized				
With 52·2 mg% Na-lactate	9	104	58	55·7	> 0·25	44	42·3
Without Na-lactate	9	116	73	62·7		69	59·4
With 500 mg% glucose	10	94	57	60·6	< 0·05	35	37·2
With 66 mg% glucose	10	118	52	44·1		9	7·6

of fertilized eggs proved to be about the same as in the control medium without lactate, and the rate of development of fertilized ova up to 48 hr after fertilization was also not affected by the absence of lactate (Table 3). The energy source in this case was probably provided by the glycolytic activity of the cultivated oviducts. This supposition was supported by an experiment in which sodium lactate as well as the other components were left in the medium, but glucose concentration was reduced from 500 to 66 mg%. In most oviducts the number of fertilized ova was actually reduced, and the first cleavage of fertilized ova was considerably retarded in all oviducts (Table 3).

The effect of pH on fertilization *in vitro* of mouse ova was observed at two regions only. The more alkaline medium, pH 7·8 to 8·1, corresponded approximately to the pH of the rabbit oviduct secretion; in the control medium at pH 6·8 to 7 the content of $NaHCO_3$ was decreased to approximately one-third.

TABLE 4

EFFECT OF pH ON FERTILIZATION RATE OF OVA AT NORMAL AND DELAYED FERTILIZATION

Time of fertilization (hr after HCG)	pH of medium	No. of oviducts	No. of ova		% ova fertilized	P
			Isolated	Fertilized		
13 to 15	7·8 to 8·1	13	114	65	57·0	>0·10
	6·7 to 7·0	13	113	72	63·3	
16 to 17	7·8 to 8·1	17	198	130	65·6	<0·025
	6·8 to 7·0	17	226	80	35·4	

TABLE 5

EFFECT OF DIFFERENT CONCENTRATIONS OF OXYGEN ON FERTILIZATION RATE OF OVA

Gaseous environment	No. of oviducts	No. of ova		% ova fertilized	P
		Isolated	Fertilized		
95% O_2, 5% CO_2	13	120	59	49·1	>0·25
95% air, 5% CO_2	13	97	48	49·4	

TABLE 6

FERTILIZATION RATE OF UTERINE SPERMATOZOA ISOLATED 1 TO 7 hr AFTER COPULATION

Sperm hr in uterus	No. of oviducts	No. of ova		% ova fertilized	P
		Isolated	Fertilized		
1 to 1½	13	143	95	66·4	<0·05
6¼ to 7	13	145	68	46·9	

Ova fertilized 16 to 17 hr after HCG injection showed significantly lower fertility in a medium of lower pH, but ova fertilized 13 to 15 hr after HCG injection showed no such effect (Table 4).

The effect of different oxygen concentrations on fertility and the initial development of zygotes was tested by fertilizing eggs *in vitro* in oviducts cultured in 5% CO_2 in either oxygen or air. The proportion of ova fertilized was approximately the same for both groups (Table 5).

The fertility of spermatozoa which were mostly agglutinated, isolated 6¼ to

7 hr after copulation, was compared with that of spermatozoa isolated 1 to 1½ hr after copulation. The results in Table 6 show a lower fertilizing capacity for spermatozoa isolated 6¼ to 7 hr after copulation. For fertilization *in vitro* it is, therefore, advisable to use spermatozoa after a shorter stay in the uterus.

Brinster & Biggers (1965) did not study the effect of different concentrations of spermatozoa on the fertilization rate of ova. Table 7 shows that concentrations in the range 300 to 4450 non-agglutinated spermatozoa/mm³ of suspension did not affect fertility.

TABLE 7

EFFECT OF DIFFERENT CONCENTRATIONS OF SPERM SUSPENSION ON FERTILITY OF OVA

No. of spermatozoa/mm³ of suspension	No. of oviducts	No. of ova		% ova fertilized
		Isolated	Fertilized	
1125	6	77	57	74·0
3037	4	44	17	38·6
3550	4	27	13	48·1
4450	3	26	18	69·2
Total high concentration	17	174	105	60·3*
550	6	55	38	69·1
790	4	20	10	50·0
300	4	16	7	43·7
560	3	29	19	65·5
Total low concentration	17	120	74	61·6*

$*P > 0.25.$

DISCUSSION

The role of lactate as energy source during the initial stages of development of zygotes was demonstrated by Whitten (1957). We found that fertilization and the initial development of mouse ova *in vitro* did not require the addition of lactate to the medium, perhaps because the glycolytic activity of the cultivated oviducts produced enough lactic acid and other metabolites from glucose to support the early stages of development of the ova. Direct proof of highly glycolytic activity of other organs in culture (lymphatic nodes, retina) was given by Lucas (1965). Decreasing the glucose concentration probably affected the metabolism of the oviducts primarily, and the composition of oviduct secretion, the process of fertilization and the first cleavages of ova secondarily. Similarly, the lack of effect of glycine on fertilization probably reflects the fact that the composition of the fluid within the cultured oviducts depends upon the activity of their cells.

It is not clear why lower pH (6·8 to 7) decreases the number of ova fertilized if fertilization is delayed. A higher pH value (7·8 to 8·1), due to a higher concentration of $NaHCO_3$, may activate metabolic processes of the gametes at fertilization directly, for example by speeding up the course of penetration, or may affect the metabolic intensity of oviduct tissues primarily and the course of the fertilizing process secondarily. The mild alkalinity of rabbit oviducts also suggests that a higher pH at fertilization is physiologically acceptable.

The difference in oxygen concentration between 5% of CO_2 in air and in oxygen had no effect on the fertilizing process, nor on the development of ova up to the blastula stage (Pavlok, 1967). Nevo (1965) showed that the critical pressure of oxygen to ensure normal respiration of bull, rabbit and cock spermatozoa is only 42 mm Hg; the concentration of oxygen in air should, therefore, be enough to support even the higher respiratory activity of uterine spermatozoa (Moundib & Chang, 1964) or fertilized ova (Sytina, 1956).

The wide range of concentration of spermatozoa shown to be optimal for fertilization of ova in explanted oviducts is consistent with the data of other authors, who have successfully used spermatozoa at concentrations from 5000 (Suzuki & Mastroiani, 1965) to 8,000,000 (Yanagimachi & Chang, 1964) spermatozoa/ml for fertilizing rabbit and hamster ova, respectively. Clots of agglutinated spermatozoa held to the end of the ampullar region *in vitro* firmly attached themselves within a minute, and when they were detached the individual spermatozoa could be observed in the orifice of the infundibulum (Pavlok, unpublished). The penetration of spermatozoa into the oviducts *in vitro* evidently depends more on the activity of the ciliated epithelium of the ampulla than on passive diffusion.

ACKNOWLEDGMENTS

The author is indebted to Dr J. Fulka and Dr V. Kopečný for their valuable advice and to Mrs L. Kracíková and Mrs M. Glasnáková for their technical assistance.

REFERENCES

AUSTIN, C. R. (1951) Observations on the penetration of sperm into the mammalian egg. *Aust. J. scient. Res.* B, **4**, 581.
AUSTIN, C. R. (1952) The 'capacitation' of the mammalian sperm. *Nature, Lond.* **170**, 326.
AUSTIN, C. R. & BISHOP, M. W. H. (1959) Differential fluorescence in living rat eggs treated with acridine orange. *Expl Cell Res.* **17**, 35.
BIGGERS, J. D., GWATKIN, R. B. L. & BRINSTER, R. L. (1962) Development of mouse embryos in organ cultures of Fallopian tubes on chemically defined medium. *Nature, Lond.* **194**, 747.
BRADEN, A. W. H. & AUSTIN, C. R. (1954) Fertilization of the mouse egg and the effect of delayed coitus and of hot-shock treatment. *Aust. J. biol. Sci.* **7**, 552.
BRINSTER, R. L. & BIGGERS, J. D. (1965) In-vitro fertilization of mouse ova within the explanted Fallopian tube. *J. Reprod. Fert.* **10**, 277.
CHANG, M. C. (1951) Fertilizing capacity of spermatozoa deposited into the Fallopian tubes. *Nature, Lond.* **168**, 697.
CHANG, M. C. (1957) A detrimental effect of seminal plasma on the fertilizing capacity of sperm. *Nature, Lond.* **179**, 258.
FISHER, R. A. & YATES, F. (1953) *Statistical tables for biological, agricultural and medical research*, 4th edn. Oliver & Boyd, Edinburgh.
GREGOIRE, A. T., GONDSKADI, D. & RAKOFF, A. (1961) The free amino acid content of the female rabbit genital tract. *Fert. Steril.* **12**, 322.
GWATKIN, R. B. L. (1962) *Discussion*. In: Symposium on Organ Culture, National Cancer Institute Monograph No. 11, p. 68. Washington.
KRZANOWSKA, H. (1966) Fertilization rate in mice after artificial insemination with epididymal 'capacitated' sperm from inbred and crossbred males. *Folia biol., Kraków*, **14**, 171.
LUCAS, D. R. (1965) Factors affecting the respiration and glycolysis of organ cultures. *Expl Cell Res.* **40**, 112.

MOUNDIB, M. S. & CHANG, M. C. (1964) Effect of in utero incubation on the metabolism of rabbit spermatozoa. *Nature, Lond.* **201,** 943.

NEVO, A. C. (1965) Dependence of sperm motility and respiration on oxygen concentration. *J. Reprod. Fert.* **9,** 103.

PAVLOK, A. (1967) Development of mouse ova in explanted oviducts: fertilization, cultivation and transplantation. *Science, N.Y.* **157,** 1457.

SUZUKI, S. & MASTROIANI, L. (1965) In vitro fertilization of rabbit ova in tubal fluid. *Am. J. Obstet. Gynec.* **93,** 465.

SYTINA, M. V. (1956) Study of oxygen absorption by rabbit's ova and zygotes. *Dokl. Vaschnil.* **9,** 11.

THIBAULT, C. & DAUZIER, L. (1960) 'Fertilisines' et fécondation in vitro de l'œuf de lapine. *C.r. hebd. Séanc. Acad. Sci., Paris,* **250,** 1358.

THIBAULT, C. & DAUZIER, L. (1961) Analyse des conditions de la fécondation in vitro de l'œuf de lapine. *Annls Biol. anim. Biochim. Biophys.* **1,** 277.

TROWELL, O. A. (1959) The culture of mature organs in a synthetic medium. *Expl Cell Res.* **16,** 118.

WHITTEN, W. K. (1957) Culture of tubal ova. *Nature, Lond.* **179,** 1081.

YANAGIMACHI, R. & CHANG, M. C. (1964) In vitro fertilization of golden hamster ova. *J. exp. Zool.* **156,** 361.

Physiological Changes in the Postnuclear Cap Region of Mammalian Spermatozoa: A Necessary Preliminary to the Membrane Fusion between Sperm and Egg Cells

R. YANAGIMACHI AND Y. D. NODA

When capacitated mammalian spermatozoa pass through the egg investments (cumulus oophorus and zona pellucida), the acrosome region of the spermatozoon undergoes profound changes to release the acrosomal contents (enzymes) (1–11, 13, 14, 17). The postnuclear cap region of the spermatozoon remains morphologically unchanged at the time of sperm capacitation and during the passage of spermatozoon through the egg investments (9–11, 17). Obviously, this part of the sperm cell is not directly involved in the mechanisms of sperm penetration through the egg investments. Its function appears to be related to the membrane fusion between sperm and egg cells (7, 10–12, 17). If the postnuclear cap region of the spermatozoon undergoes no changes whatsoever at the time of sperm capacitation, both uncapacitated and capacitated spermatozoa should be equally able to enter the eggs if they are brought directly to the plasma membrane of the egg. The present experiments were designed to determine whether this is the case.

MATERIALS AND METHODS

Adult females of the golden hamster (*Mesocricetus auratus*) were treated with pregnant mare serum and human chorionic gonadotropin and killed between 15 and 16 hours after HCG injection (about 1–5 hours after ovulation; 15). The oviducts were excised and flushed with Tyrode's solution. The eggs were freed from cumulus cells by treatment with 0.1%

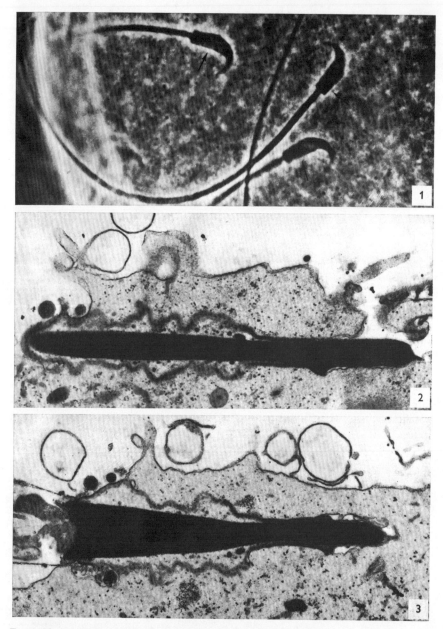

FIG. 1. Phase-contrast micrograph of capacitated spermatozoa 15 minutes after insemination. Arrows indicate the postnuclear cap regions of spermatozoa. × 1700.

FIGS. 2 and 3. Electron micrographs of a capacitated spermatozoon (two serial, sagittal sections of the same spermatozoon) 15 minutes after insemination. × 17,000.

bovine testicular hyaluronidase (Nutritional Biochemicals Corp.) in Tyrode's solution for 8–10 minutes at 25–30°C. The zona pellucida was dissolved by immersing the eggs in 0.1% trypsin (1–300, Nutritional Biochem. Corp.) in Tyrode's solution for 3–4 minutes at 25–30°C. The "naked" eggs were transferred into a mixture of detoxified bovine follicular fluid (16) and Tyrode's solution (1:1) and kept there for 20 minutes or less (at 30–37°C).

The spermatozoa were capacitated by mixing equal volumes (0.05 ml) of epididymal sperm suspension (1 to 2×10^7 sperms per milliliter of Tyrode's solution) and detoxified bovine follicular fluid under mineral oil in a watch glass, and incubating for 3 hours at 37–38°C. Since hamster spermatozoa are not capacitated under such conditions before 2 hours (16), those which were incubated for only 10 minutes or less were considered uncapacitated. The "naked" eggs which had been kept in the bovine follicular fluid solution were transferred (accompanied by about 0.05 ml of the solution) into the suspensions of capacitated and uncapacitated spermatozoa under the oil. After having been incubated for 15–60 minutes at 37–38°C, the eggs were mounted between a slide and coverslip and examined with a phase-contrast microscope (100×10) for evidence of sperm penetration. The eggs were also examined by electron microscopy using the techniques described previously (17).

RESULTS

When the eggs were examined 1 hour after insemination with capacitated spermatozoa, 100% of them (a total of 81 eggs in 10 experiments) were found to be penetrated by spermatozoa. The cortical granules of the eggs had completely disappeared, and the egg nuclei were at the late telophase of the second maturation division or in the early pronuclear stage. The second polar body was always extruded. The majority of the eggs were polyspermic, and several swelling sperm heads were often found within one egg. In many cases, more than ten enlarged sperm heads were seen in one egg.

The results were entirely different when the eggs were inseminated with uncapacitated spermatozoa. None of the eggs (a total of 62 eggs in 8 experiments) was found penetrated by spermatozoa at 1 hour after insemination, despite the presence of numerous spermatozoa adhering to their surfaces.

FIGS. 4 and 5. Phase-contrast micrographs of capacitated spermatozoa 30 minutes (Fig. 4) and 60 minutes (Fig. 5) after insemination. × 1700.

FIGS. 6 and 7. Electron micrographs of the heads of capacitated spermatozoa 30 minutes (Fig. 6) and 60 minutes (Fig. 7) after insemination. Fig. 6, × 17,000; Fig. 7, × 11,000.

FIGS. 8 and 9. Phase-contrast micrographs of uncapacitated spermatozoa 60 minutes after insemination. Arrows indicate motionless (dead) spermatozoa. Note that cortical granules of the egg remain intact. × 1700.

FIGS. 10 and 11. Electron micrographs of uncapacitated spermatozoa 60 minutes after insemination. Microvilli of the eggs surround the sperm heads, but the spermatozoa are not incorporated with the eggs. × 14,000.

FIG. 12. Electron micrograph of a dead spermatozoon on the surface of an egg 60 minutes after insemination. Note that both head and detached acrosome cap (arrow) of the dead spermatozoon are surrounded by microvilli of the egg. × 9500.

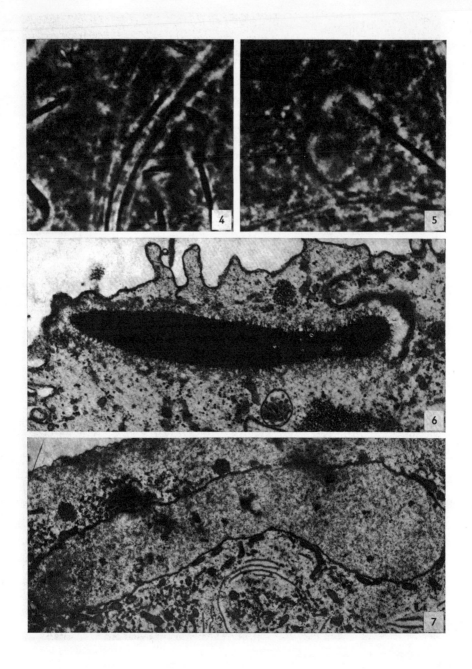

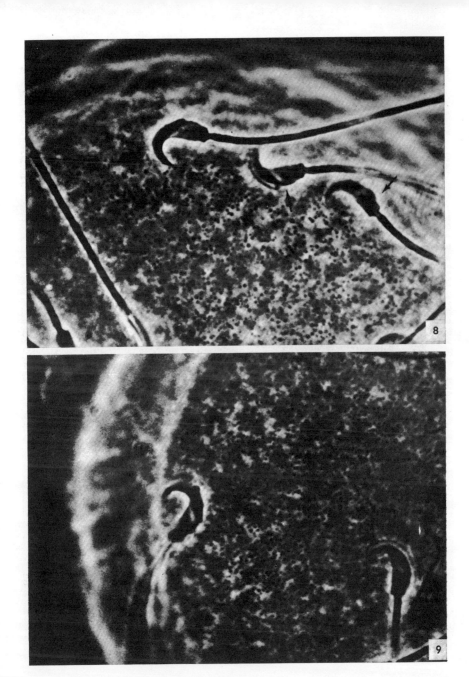

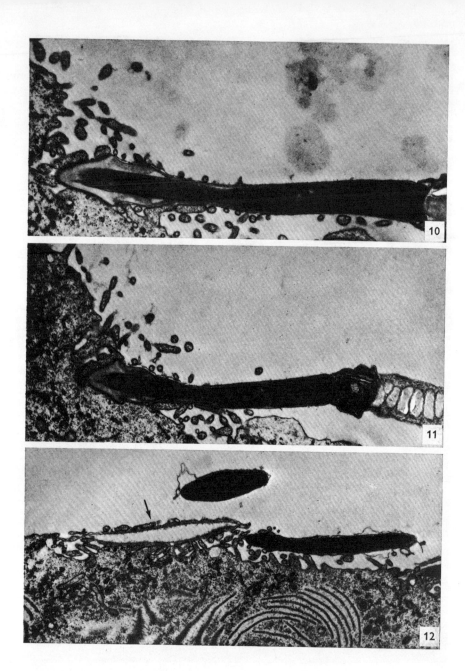

Figs. 1–3 show phase-contrast and electron micrographs of capacitated spermatozoa at 15 minutes after insemination. It will be seen that the membrane fusion between sperm and egg cells is completed at the postnuclear cap region of the spermatozoon, and the sperm nucleus has begun to disperse in that region. At 30–60 minutes after insemination, the heads (nuclei) of the capacitated spermatozoa were completely within the egg cytoplasm and were extensively swollen (Figs. 4–7).

Figs. 8–12 show phase-contrast and electron micrographs of uncapacitated spermatozoa at 60 minutes after insemination. Obviously, the spermatozoa are still outside the eggs and there is no indication of membrane fusion between sperm and egg cells. On many occasions motionless (dead) spermatozoa were found attached to the surface of the eggs. In most of them, the acrosome cap, together with the overlying plasma membrane, was detaching or had been detached (Figs. 8 and 9). No such dead spermatozoa were found incorporated with the eggs (Fig. 12).

CONCLUSION AND COMMENT

A conclusion to be drawn from these observations is that although the postnuclear cap region of the spermatozoon does not manifest any visible morphological change at the time of capacitation, it certainly undergoes some important physiological change which is an essential preliminary to membrane fusion between sperm and egg cells. We would like to emphasize that *capacitation* not only enables the spermatozoon to penetrate the egg investments, but also enables it to be incorporated with the egg itself.

At the present time, it is not known whether the physiological changes in the postnuclear cap region of the spermatozoon are provoked only in the plasma membrane or in both the plasma membrane and the postnuclear cap itself. The only thing certain from the present study is that the physiological properties of the plasma membrane of the postnuclear cap region of the spermatozoon change markedly at the time of sperm capacitation.

The authors wish to express their sincere thanks to Dr. R. W. Noyes and Dr. J. C. Dan for their helpful suggestions. This work was supported by grants from U.S. Public Health Service (HD-03402), the Ford Foundation, and the Population Council.

REFERENCES

1. Austin, C. R., *Nature* **181**, 851 (1958).
2. —— *J. Reprod. Fertility* **6**, 313 (1963).
3. —— *Proc. 5th Intern. Congr. Animal Reprod. Trento* Vol. II, p. 7 (1964).
4. —— *Intern. J. Fertility* **12**, 25 (1967).

5. AUSTIN, C. R. and BISHOP, M. W. H., *Proc. Roy. Soc.* **B149**, 241 (1958).
6. BARROS, C., BEDFORD, J. M., FRANKLIN, L. E. and AUSTIN, C. R., *J. Cell Biol.* **34**, C 1 (1967).
7. BARROS, C. and FRANKLIN, L. E., *J. Cell Biol.* **37**, C 13 (1968).
8. BEDFORD, J. M., *J. Reprod. Fertility, Suppl.* 2, 35 (1967).
9. —— *Am. J. Anat.* **123**, 329 (1968).
10. PIKO, L., *Intern. J. Fertility* **12**, 377 (1967).
11. PIKO, L. and TYLER, A., *Proc. 5th Intern. Congr. Animal Reprod. Trento* Vol. II, p. 372 (1964).
12. STEFANINI, M., OURA, C. and ZAMBONI, L., *J. Submicroscop. Cytol.* **1**, 1 (1969).
13. YANAGIMACHI, R., *Proc. 5th Intern. Congr. Animal Reprod. Trento* Vol. III, p. 321 (1964).
14. —— *J. Reprod. Fertility* **11**, 359 (1966).
15. —— *ibid.* **18**, 275 (1969).
16. —— *J. Exptl. Zool.* **170**, 269 (1969).
17. YANAGIMACHI, R. and NODA, Y. D., *J. Ultrastruct. Res.* **31**, 465 (1970).

Biochemical Aspects of Early Mammalian Embryogenesis In Vitro

INCORPORATION OF CARBON FROM GLUCOSE AND PYRUVATE INTO THE PREIMPLANTATION MOUSE EMBRYO

R. L. BRINSTER

It has been shown that the early stages of the mouse embryo oxidize pyruvate to a much greater extent than glucose [6, 7]. After blastocyst formation, the embryo oxidizes glucose as well as pyruvate. Pyruvate appears to be the central energy source for the two-cell embryo, for the fertilized zygote, and for the oocyte [1, 3, 4, 6, 7]. Glucose will not support the development of the mouse embryo before the four-cell stage, but the embryos develop well after the eight-cell stage when glucose is the only energy source. Work done on the uptake of glucose and pyruvate suggests that the uptake of pyruvate is greater than the uptake of glucose at the one-cell stage but not at the two-cell stage [13, 15]. The question arises whether pyruvate carbon is also incorporated into the embryo to a greater extent than glucose carbon during the first few cleavages.

One possible site for incorporation of the carbon accumulated by the embryo would be in the glycogen of the embryo. Histochemical studies have shown that there is considerable glycogen in the embryo at ovulation and that there is an increase in embryo glycogen from the one-cell to the two-cell stage. There is almost a complete disappearance of the glycogen during the blastocyst stage [12]. Biochemical studies have shown very little glycogen present at ovulation, but a large amount of glycogen is accumulated from the one-cell to the eight-cell stage [10].

The studies reported here were designed to determine the incorporation of carbon from glucose and pyruvate into the successive preimplantation stages of the mouse embryo. An attempt was made to identify the fraction of the embryo into which the incorporation occurred.

METHODS

Embryos were obtained from eight-week-old random-bred Swiss female mice, which were superovulated and mated with Swiss males. The method of collecting and handling the embryos and the formula of the

Table 1. *Culture medium*

Component	G/l	mM
NaCl	6.975	119.32
KCl	0.356	4.78
CaCl$_2$	0.189	1.71
KH$_2$PO$_4$	0.162	1.19
MgSO$_4$7H$_2$O	0.294	1.19
NaHCO$_3$	2.106	25.07
Glucose	1.000	5.56
Pyruvate	0.055	0.50
Penicillin G	100 U/ml	—
Streptomycin sulfate	50 μg/ml	—
Crystalline bovine Serum albumin	1.000	—

medium used during preliminary manipulations have been described [2, 8]. Cumulus cells were removed from the one-cell embryo with hyaluronidase at a concentration of 300 units/ml [5]. Before the embryos were placed in the experimental medium, they were washed three times by sequential transfer, in a volume of 5 μl, through three changes of medium (3 ml). They were then placed in small drops (50 μl) of culture medium under paraffin oil as described by Brinster [2]. The formula of the culture medium is shown in table 1. Only the pyruvate *or* the glucose was radioactive. The specific activity of the radioactive pyruvate and glucose was 16.6 and 3.0 mC/mmole respectively. The embryos were incubated 20–24 h and then removed to assay radioactivity.

In the few experiments where only total activity per embryo was measured, the method used was similar to that previously described [13, 14]. The external radioactivity was removed from the embryos by centrifugation in a 2.6 ml Pichler-Spikes centrifuge tube (Kimble 45156) with a capillary tip (bore 2 mm). The bottom 0.5 cm of the tip was filled with 10 % w/v sucrose solution containing 1 % v/v formalin, and the remaining capillary portion of the tube was filled with isotonic sucrose. Above this, the wide portion of the tube was filled with approximately 1.5 ml of non-radioactive culture medium. After incubation the embryos were picked up in approx. 5 μl of medium and placed in the top of the tube. The tube was immediately centrifuged at 500 g for 3 min. After centrifugation the culture medium was removed, the inner surface of the tube was wiped dry, rinsed with 1 ml of non-radioactive medium and again wiped dry. The sucrose column was carefully removed, beginning at the top of the column, to within 1 cm of the bottom. The next 0.5 cm of sucrose was removed and placed in a scintillation vial to act as a background count for the embryo. The bottom of the tube was then removed and transferred with its contents to a scintillation vial. One ml of 1 M hyamine and 10 ml of scintillation fluid were added to the vial.

In most of the experiments the embryos were recovered after incubation and transferred in 2 μl through three successive washes of the medium shown in table 1 in which the substrates were not radioactive.

The embryos were then transferred in 5 μl of the final wash to a 2 ml centrifuge tube containing 100 μl of water to cause lysis of the embryo cells. The tube was frozen and thawed three times and was agitated on a mixer during each thawing to assure complete breakdown of the cytoplasmic structure. One mg of bovine serum albumin and 1 mg of glycogen in 20 μl of water were added to the tube to act as cold carrier. One hundred μl of 10 % trichloroacetic acid (TCA) was added to the tubes, the contents mixed, and the tube centrifuged (1000 g for 3 min). The supernatant was drawn off and saved, and the precipitate was resuspended in 200 μl of 5 % TCA. The tube was centrifuged (1000 g for 3 min), and the supernatant was drawn off and added to the first supernatant. The precipitate was dissolved in 100 μl of 10 % KOH and placed in a scintillation vial. One ml of Beckman Biosolve no. 1 and 10 ml of scintillation fluid were added to the vial. To the approx. 400 μl of supernatant drawn off during the above procedure, 600 μl of 95 % ethyl alcohol was added. These were mixed and centrifuged. The precipitate was washed again in 95 % alcohol and aliquots of the supernatant fluid were saved for scintillation counting. The precipitate was dissolved in 100 μl of water and prepared for counting as described for the precipitate above.

In the third group of experiments the alcohol precipitate was dissolved in 0.5 ml of 1 M acetic acid buffer (pH 2.5) and was subjected to column chromatography to identify further the composition of this component. The columns were prepared from Pasteur pipettes and are shown in fig. 1. The acetic acid, containing the dissolved precipitate, was put on a column containing 300–400 mg of Dowex 1-X8 anionic exchange resin. The effluent of the first column was immediately put on a column containing 300–400 mg (w/w) of Dowex 50W-X8 cationic exchange resin. The acetic acid containing the dissolved precipitate was followed by five 1 ml washes of acetic acid. The anionic column was then washed with five 1 ml washes of 1 N HCl, and the cationic column was washed with five 1 ml washes of 1 N NaOH. All the washes were

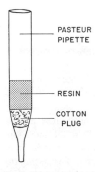

PASTEUR PIPETTE

RESIN

COTTON PLUG

Fig. 1. Column used to separate components of mouse embryo. The column consists of a portion of a Pasteur pipette containing a cotton plug and 300–400 mg of resin.

Table 2. *Carbon accumulated from glucose and pyruvate by the two-cell mouse embryo*

	Substrate concentration			
Pyruvate = Glucose =	5×10^{-4} M[a] 1.0 mg/ml	5×10^{-4} M 1.0 mg/ml[a]	5×10^{-4} M[a] 0.1 mg/ml	5×10^{-4} M 0.1 mg/ml[a]
Experiment	$\mu\mu$ Atoms of carbon accumulated per embryo/h			
1	0.604	1.881	0.657	0.714
2	0.696	2.116	0.591	1.297
3	0.561	1.179	0.522	0.574
4	0.671	1.812	0.577	0.587
5	0.595	1.358	0.737	1.175
6	0.591	1.785	0.644	0.413
Mean ± S.E.	0.621 ± 0.040	1.689 ± 0.240	0.621 ± 0.050	0.793 ± 0.241

[a] Indicates radioactive substrate; labelled substrates were uniformly labelled ^{14}C.

saved for radioactivity determinations. The washes, except the NaOH, were placed in 1 ml volumes in scintillation vials, dried, and suspended with Beckman Biosolve no. 1 and 10 ml of scintillation fluid for counting. The scintillation fluid contained 0.5 % (w/v) 2,5-diphenyloxazole (PPO) and 0.03 % (w/v), 1,4-bis-2 (4-methyl-5-phenyloxazolylbenzene (M$_2$POPOP) in toluene. This was the scintillation fluid used in all experiments except with the NaOH washes which were suspended in 10 ml of a solution containing 80 g Cabosil, 252 g naphthalene, 300 mg M$_2$POPOP, 14 g PPO, 200 ml absolute ethyl alcohol, and 1800 ml dioxane.

RESULTS

In the first experiments total uptake of substrate by the embryo over a 20 h period beginning at the two-cell stage was examined. The medium contained both pyruvate and glucose, but only one substrate was radioactive in each experimental treatment. The experimental treatments and the results are shown in table 2. The accumulation of carbon from glucose is approximately three times greater than carbon accumulation from pyruvate when the concentration of glucose in the medium is 1 mg/ml. Even when the concentration of glucose in the medium is only 0.1 mg/ml, more glucose carbon than pyruvate carbon is accumulated by the two-cell embryo. Decreasing the concentration of glucose in the medium from 1.0 to 0.1 mg/ml has no effect on pyruvate carbon accumulation by the embryo.

In the second group of experiments, carbon accumulation by the embryo from glucose and pyruvate was examined throughout the entire preimplantation period. The experimental treatments and the results are shown in table 3. The carbon accumulated in each of three fractions was measured. The TCA precipitate was considered to be mostly protein with some other macromolecules such as nucleic acids. The ethyl alcohol precipitate of the TCA supernatant was considered to be primarily glycogen. The ethyl alcohol supernatant contained all the rest of the carbon accumulated by the embryo. The most striking observation is that carbon from glucose is accumulated by the embryo to a much greater extent than carbon from pyruvate throughout the preimplantation period. Another important observation is the sharp increase in carbon accumulation in the morula and blastocyst stage of development. This increase is mostly from glucose carbon. There appears to be very little carbon accumulated from exogenous glucose or pyruvate into glycogen (ETOH precipitate) in the early stages of development. From the blastocysts, however, the ethyl alcohol precipitate fraction contains a considerable amount of carbon from exogenous glucose.

Table 3. *Carbon accumulation in mouse embryos*

Growth period	Carbon accumulated			
	Protein (TCA ppt)	Glycogen (ETOH ppt)	ETOH Supernatant	Total
A. *Carbon accumulated from radioactive pyruvate by mouse embryos*				
1-cell to 2-cell	0.279 ± 0.006	0.004 ± 0.001	0.479 ± 0.022	0.761 ± 0.027
2-cell to 4-cell	0.258 ± 0.028	0.004 ± 0.001	0.425 ± 0.048	0.686 ± 0.073
8-cell to morula	0.665 ± 0.009	0.006 ± 0.001	0.573 ± 0.022	1.244 ± 0.036
Morula to blastocyst	0.869 ± 0.042	0.010 ± 0.003	0.914 ± 0.059	1.793 ± 0.064
B. *Carbon accumulated from radioactive glucose by mouse embryos*				
1-cell to 2-cell	1.114 ± 0.048	0.018 ± 0.002	0.527 ± 0.013	1.648 ± 0.036
2-cell to 4-cell	1.072 ± 0.115	0.020 ± 0.006	0.628 ± 0.024	1.719 ± 0.126
8-cell to morula	2.657 ± 0.161	2.912 ± 0.077	1.443 ± 0.137	7.012 ± 0.671
Morula to blastocyst	3.372 ± 0.091	14.020 ± 1.264	2.617 ± 0.114	20.008 ± 1.378

Carbon accumulated is given in $\mu\mu$ atoms of carbon/embryo/h, and each value is the mean of 4 determinations.
Embryos cultured approximately 24 h in medium containing both pyruvate (5×10^{-4} M) and glucose (1 mg/ml). Only one of the substrates was labelled in each experiment.

The ethyl alcohol precipitate fraction from blastocysts was examined further by column chromatography to determine whether this fraction contained substances other than glycogen. The results of the column chromatography of this fraction are shown in table 4. The uncharged molecules in the acetic acid at pH 2.5 (probably glycogen) were not adsorbed to either resin and appear in the acetic acid wash. This is about 60 % of the total carbon accumulation from glucose. The HCl wash of the anionic resin includes those compounds which were negatively charged at pH 2.5 (probably small nucleotides) and were adsorbed to the anionic resin. Very little of the accumulated carbon is in this subfraction.

The NaOH wash of the cationic resin includes those compounds which were positively charged at pH 2.5 (probably amino acids and peptides) and were adsorbed to the cationic resin. A considerable amount of the carbon from glucose is in this subfraction.

DISCUSSION

In the studies by Wales & Brinster [13] the uptake rate for glucose carbon by the two-cell mouse embryo was 2.87 $\mu\mu$moles of carbon/embryo/30 min. In the present study the average rate of incorporation for the same age embryo was 1.689 $\mu\mu$moles of carbon/embryo/h. Although there are some tech-

Table 4. *Separation by column chromatography of ethyl alcohol precipitate fraction of carbon accumulated from radioactive glucose by the mouse morula*

Effluent	Carbon accumulated in $\mu\mu$ atoms/embryo/h				
	Expt 1	Expt 2	Expt 3	Mean	%
Acetic acid wash through both resins	3.332	3.492	4.842	3.889	59.7
HCl wash of anionic resin	0.006	0.033	0.013	0.017	0.3
NaOH wash of cationic resin	2.259	1.974	3.581	2.605	40.0

Table 5. *Comparison of pyruvate and glucose carbon utilization by the mouse embryo*

| | $\mu\mu$ atoms of carbon/embryo/h | | | | | |
| | From pyruvate | | | From glucose | | |
Stage of development	Average CO_2 produced [7]	Carbon incor-porated	Total	Average CO_2 produced [6]	Carbon incor-porated	Total
1-cell to 2-cell	6.490	0.761	7.251	0.935	1.684	2.619
2-cell to 8-cell	6.640	0.686	7.326	1.675	1.719	3.394
8-cell to morula	9.605	1.244	10.849	5.550	7.012	12.562
Morula to blastocyst	13.845	1.793	15.638	11.765	20.008	31.773

In studies on CO_2 production, only one substrate was in the medium; therefore, these values set maximum values for the particular substrate and are not necessarily additive.

nical differences between the two studies, such as the incubation time and the inclusion of pyruvate in the medium used in the present study, the difference between the values (approx. 2 $\mu\mu$moles/embryo/30 min) probably represents the initial rapid accumulation of labelled intermediates in glucose metabolism by the embryo. In the longer studies, these labelled intermediates which are accumulated first represent only a small amount of the final calculated hourly rate.

The data in table 3 show that at every developmental stage glucose carbon is incorporated into each of the fractions to a greater extent than is pyruvate. This is a somewhat surprising result in view of the dependency of the early stages of the mouse embryo before the four-cell stage on pyruvate for development. In addition, we know that the two-cell mouse embryo will develop into a blastocyst in vitro in a medium containing only pyruvate. This suggests that despite the incorporation of more carbon from glucose than from pyruvate into the embryo, it is the oxidation of pyruvate which is essential for the development of the embryo. Table 5 shows the relative rates of oxidation and incorporation for the two substrates, and the

data suggest that oxidation rather than incorporation accounts for most of the carbon used by the embryo up to the morula stage. From the morula through blastocyst development, carbon incorporation is greater than carbon oxidation.

There is a considerable amount of glycogen in the mouse embryo [12], and it has been suggested that most of this glycogen is synthesized by the embryo between the one-cell stage and the eight-cell stage [10]. The biochemical studies show an increase of 2.1 mμg of glycogen per embryo during the 48 h developmental period from the one-cell to the eight-cell stage [10]. The studies reported here on incorporation of pyruvate and glucose into the embryo during this period of development indicate that about 0.023 $\mu\mu$ atoms/h of carbon from these substrates is incorporated into the glycogen of the embryo. To form 2.1 mμg of glycogen in 48 h would require the accumulation of 1.46 $\mu\mu$ atoms of carbon per hour per embryo. Thus, carbon from pyruvate and glucose incorporated into glycogen can account for only about 1.6% of the required amount. The rest of the carbon must come from other sources (perhaps endogenous protein) or from precursors which might give a positive histochemical test and not be detected biochemically. Another possibility is that glycogen synthesis does not occur under the in vitro conditions of the incorporation studies but does occur in vivo.

The very large incorporation of glucose into the ethyl alcohol precipitate fraction during blastocyst formation is surprising, since it is during this period when the histochemical studies show that the glycogen content of the embryo is decreasing. Closer examination of this fraction indicates that about 40 % of it has chromatographic characteristics similar to amino acids and peptides. It would not be surprising to find in the developing blastocyst a large pool of amino acids and peptides being formed since we know this is a period of active protein synthesis [9, 11]. The incorporation of glucose carbon into the other 60 % of the fraction indicates that glycogen is actively synthesized as well as utilized during this period. Utilization must be greater than synthesis if the histochemical studies on glycogen content are correct.

Financial support for this work came from National Institutes of Health grants HD 03071 and HD 02315. The expert technical assistance of Miss Mary Ryans is gratefully acknowledged.

REEERENCES

1. Biggers, J D, Whittingham, D G & Donahue, R P, Proc natl acad sci US 58 (1967) 560.
2. Brinster R L, Exptl cell res 32 (1963) 205.
3. — J exptl zool 158 (1965) 59.
4. — J reprod fertil 10 (1965) 227.
5. — Biochim biophys acta 10 (1965) 439.
6. — Exptl cell res 47 (1967) 271.
7. — Ibid 47 (1967) 634.
8. — The mammalian oviduct (ed E S E Hafez & R Blandau) p. 419. University of Chicago, New York (1969).
9. Mintz, B, J exptl zool 156 (1964) 85.
10. Stern, S & Biggers, J D, J exptl zool 168 (1968) 61.
11. Tasca, R J, RNA synthesis and protein synthesis in preimplantation stage mouse embryos, Ph.D. thesis. Temple University, Philadelphia, Pa (1969).
12. Thomson, J L & Brinster, R L, Anat rec 155 (1966) 97.
13. Wales, R G & Brinster, R L, J reprod fertil 15 (1968) 415.
14. Wales, R G & O'Shea, T, Austr j biol sci 19 (1966) 167.
15. Wales, R G & Whittingham, D G, Biochim biophys acta 148 (1967) 703.

105

RADIOACTIVE CARBON DIOXIDE PRODUCTION FROM PYRUVATE
AND LACTATE BY THE PREIMPLANTATION RABBIT EMBRYO

R. L. BRINSTER

The mouse embryo, during the first few days of development, oxidizes glucose to carbon dioxide in only small quantities [4]. The ability of the embryo to oxidize glucose gradually increases during the preimplantation period and reaches a maximum at the time of implantation. However, it has been shown that the embryo can readily oxidize pyruvate and lactate to CO_2 at the time of ovulation as well as during the entire preimplantation period [5]. These studies confirmed the preference and, indeed, dependence of the early mouse embryo on pyruvate and perhaps on lactate as an energy source. The importance of pyruvate and lactate to the embryo had previously been suggested by in vitro culture studies showing that the 2-cell embryo would develop in a medium containing only pyruvate or lactate as an energy source, but not in one containing only glucose [3].

Recent studies on the preimplantation rabbit embryo have shown that the oxidation of glucose to carbon dioxide in this species is also low at the time of ovulation but that the ability to oxidize glucose gradually increases during the preimplantation period to a maximum at implantation. The pattern is similar to that seen in the mouse embryo. This was somewhat unexpected

for two reasons. First, the early rabbit embryo has been readily cultivated in vitro in a variety of media having glucose as the major energy source, suggesting that glucose could act as an energy source; and second, the mouse embryo was shown to have 60 times as much lactate dehydrogenase activity as the rabbit embryo, suggesting that this enzyme might be functionally of more significance to the mouse embryo than to the rabbit embryo [2, 6].

The investigation was undertaken to study the formation of carbon dioxide from pyruvate and lactate by the preimplantation rabbit embryo, and thus to be able to compare the mouse and rabbit embryo in respect to their ability to oxidize these energy sources and glucose during the preimplantation period.

MATERIALS AND METHODS

Rabbit embryos were obtained by superovulating female New Zealand White rabbits. The rabbits were obtained from a single commercial source and weighed 3 to 3.5 kg. Unfertilized, fertilized and cleavage-stage embryos were obtained by superovulation as previously described [7]. An average of 30 embryos from each female were obtained by the methods employed.

Embryos of different developmental stages were flushed from the reproductive tract of the females at appropriate times after mating and ovulation. Eagles medium contain-

106

Table 1. *Radioactive carbon dioxide produced from lactate by the preimplantation rabbit embryo*

Stage of development	Molar concentration of lactate					
	1×10^{-1}	5×10^{-2}	1×10^{-2}	5×10^{-3}	1×10^{-3}	5×10^{-4}
Unfertilized	31.40 ± 8.22 (5)	14.71 ± 2.85 (5)	12.75 ± 1.74 (4)	4.79 ± 0.43 (5)	3.24 ± 0.19 (4)	2.03 ± 0.53 (4)
Fertilized	26.91 ± 8.24 (8)	11.28 ± 1.84 (9)	11.44 ± 4.82 (6)	5.73 ± 0.97 (6)	1.71 ± 0.20 (4)	1.14 ± 0.11 (5)
Day 2	32.99 ± 9.32 (5)	22.11 ± 7.71 (8)	9.23 ± 2.45 (7)	4.69 ± 1.04 (7)	2.12 ± 0.29 (4)	1.25 ± 0.40 (4)
3	35.20 ± 7.79 (4)	23.06 ± 2.53 (5)	21.88 ± 4.23 (5)	9.97 ± 1.49 (7)	3.40 ± 0.38 (4)	1.57 ± 0.63 (4)
4	232.9 ± 42.8 (8)	178.2 ± 46.0 (5)	47.6 ± 10.1 (4)	34.4 ± 8.9 (4)	11.8 ± 3.1 (4)	2.86 ± 0.8 (4)
	1090.8 ± 199.0 (5)	655.2 ± 55.3 (5)	451.4 ± 115.0 (7)	329.1 ± 67.5 (5)	51.0 ± 11.4 (5)	48.9 ± 13.5 (5)
6	5750.2 ± 1368.5 (4)	3844.3 ± 662.0 (4)	2156.5 ± 476.4 (5)	762.3 ± 154.1 (4)	247.9 ± 79.0 (4)	130.4 ± 35.4 (4)

All values are $\mu\mu$moles of CO_2 produced/embryo/h ± S.E.M.
The number of determinations are in parentheses.

ng 10 % fetal calf serum was used to flush the embryos from the reproductive tract and for storing the embryos during the collection period. When sufficient embryos were collected, they were washed 3 times in a modified Krebs-Ringer bicarbonate solution containing no energy substrates [4]. From the last wash, the embryos were placed in the incubation medium containing the radioactive substrate.

The system used for growing the embryos in the radioactive medium and the method for extracting the CO_2 have been described previously [4]. The culture medium used was similar to that used for washing the embryos but with radioactive pyruvate and lactate added. The ^{14}C-L-lactate was universly labelled, with a specific activity of 0.1–0.2 mc/mmole and was obtained from Calbiochem. The ^{14}C-pyruvate was universly labelled, with a specific activity of 1.0–2.0 mc/mmole, and was obtained from Nuclear Chicago. The isotope was diluted with cold substrate to obtain the desired final concentration. All concentrations of lactate are for DL-lactate unless specified L-lactate. The DL-lactate is 50 % L-lactate. Sodium lactate or sodium pyruvate are substituted for NaCl in the culture medium to obtain the desired concentration. Osmolarity is maintained at 0.3C8 and pH at 7.38 [3]. The volume of the incubation medium was 100 μl in all cases and the incubation time was 4 h except for day-5 and day-6 embryos. For these embryos, which are quite large, the incubation time was 1 h and $\frac{1}{2}$ h respectively.

RESULTS

In the first studies, sodium lactate was employed at different concentrations as the only energy source in the culture medium. Six concentrations ranging from 5×10^{-4} M to 1×10^{-1} M were used, based on information available from studies on mouse embryos [3, 5]. The specific activity of the lactate was the same at all concentrations. The concentrations used and the amount of CO_2 formed at each concentration are shown in table 1.

Carbon dioxide production from labelled lactate increased with lactate concentration in the medium and with developmental age of the embryo. The increase in CO_2 production does not seem to be linearly related to concentration, since the increment in CO_2 production due to lactate concentration decreases as the concentration increases. In addition, a 10-fold increase in concentration of lactate does not result in a 10-fold increase in CO_2 production. The data seems to indicate no obvious optimum lactate concentration for CO_2 production. However, in general the effects of developmental stage of the embryo on CO_2 formation seem to be similar for all the concentrations of lactate examined.

The effect of the developmental stage on CO_2 production is not obvious up through day 2. After day 2, there is an increase in CO_2 production during each 24 h period of development. The magnitude of the increment for each 24 h period increases with the age of the embryo. The large increases between days 4 and 5 and

Table 2. *Radioactive carbon dioxide produced from pyruvate by the preimplantation rabbit embryo*

Stage of development	Molar concentration of pyruvate				
	5×10^{-3}	1×10^{-3}	5×10^{-4}	1×10^{-4}	5×10^{-5}
Unfertilized	19.92± 0.85 (5)	16.33± 1.22 (4)	16.68± 0.86 (5)	9.40± 0.45 (4)	6.41± 0.46 (4)
Fertilized	13.31± 0.98 (4)	16.53± 1.23 (5)	14.47± 0.55 (5)	9.87± 0.54 (4)	5.60± 1.06 (4)
Day 2	13.73± 1.36 (4)	14.20± 0.72 (4)	13.42± 1.22 (4)	6.79± 0.31 (4)	5.51± 0.28 (4)
3	28.24± 3.12 (4)	25.47± 1.46 (4)	22.31± 1.34 (4)	10.05± 0.89 (4)	5.76± 0.33 (4)
4	210.18± 17.32 (4)	228.29± 30.20 (4)	201.19± 25.86 (6)	52.00± 5.52 (4)	42.52± 0.85 (4)
5	3179.6 ± 565.7 (4)	2208.0 ± 305.6 (4)	2032.9 ± 331.7 (5)	782.1 ± 90.4 (4)	493.6 ± 68.1 (4)
6	20573.0 ±2814.0 (4)	10585.0 ±2713.0 (5)	9882.0 ±1439.0 (5)	3095.0 ±415.0 (4)	2515.0 ±594.0 (4)

All values are $\mu\mu$moles of CO_2 produced/embryo/h ± S.E.M.
The number of determinations are in parentheses.

days 5 and 6 are a direct result of the rapid increase which takes place in the tissue mass during this period.

In the second group of studies, sodium pyruvate was employed at different concentrations as the only energy source in the medium. In this case, 5 concentrations ranging from 5×10^{-5} M to 5×10^{-3} M were used, and the concentrations were again chosen on the basis of previous work done with mouse embryos. [3]. The specific activity of the pyruvate was the same at all concentrations. The concentrations used and the results are shown in table 2.

Carbon dioxide production increased with increasing pyruvate concentrations up to 5×10^{-4} M, but the increases did not appear to be linearly related to concentration. Above a concentration of 5×10^{-4} M, there was very little if any increase in CO_2 formation in the early developmental stages, and only small increases on days 4 and 5. This suggests that 5×10^{-4} M represents an optimum concentration of pyruvate for CO_2 production.

There is very little effect of developmental stage on CO_2 production from pyruvate during the first 2 days of the rabbit embryo's life. Then, between day 2 and 3 there is an approximate doubling of CO_2 production. After day 3, the rise in CO_2 production is dramatic, similar to the findings for lactate, and is probably a direct result of the increase in tissue mass.

DISCUSSION

In the case of CO_2 production from pyruvate there appeared to be an optimum concentration for CO_2 production at 5×10^{-4} M. This is the same optimum concentration of pyruvate which has been found for the development of 2-cell mouse embryos [3]. An optimum lactate concentration for CO_2 production was not clearly obvious from the data. There is some suggestion that the rate of increase in CO_2 production decreases between 1×10^{-2} M and 1×10^{-1} M, and this may suggest that an optimum exists in this range. In the early mouse embryo, the optimum concentration for development has been found to be 5×10^{-2} M, and in the absence of further information 5×10^{-2} M lactate has been used in the following discussion as a tentative optimum for lactate concentration for the early rabbit embryo.

One of the most striking conclusions resulting from the results reported here is the similarity in energy source utilization between the early mouse embryo and the early rabbit embryo. In table 3

Table 3. *Comparison of carbon dioxide production from glucose, pyruvate and lactate for preimplantation mouse and rabbit embryos*

Stage of development	Glucose		Pyruvate		Lactate	
	Mouse	Rabbit	Mouse	Rabbit	Mouse	Rabbit
Unfertilized	0.13	0.61	7.24	16.68	3.09	14.71
Fertilized	0.68	0.81	6.95	14.47	3.31	11.28
Day						
2	1.19	5.98	6.03	13.42	2.77	22.11
3	2.16	13.71	7.25	22.31	4.54	23.06
4	8.84	50.33	11.96	201.2	11.20	178.2
5	14.69	1335.15	15.73	2032.9	15.06	655.2
6	—	4904.98	—	9882.3	—	3844.3

All values are $\mu\mu$moles of CO_2 produced/embryo/h.
The substrate concentration was for glucose, 1 mg/ml; for pyruvate, 5×10^{-4} M; and for lactate, 5×10^{-2} M. The glucose values for the rabbit are from Brinster [7], and the values for the mouse are from Brinster [4, 5].

there is a summary of this information. In considering the data in the table, two things should be kept in mind. First the ovulated rabbit ovum is approx. 3.5 times the volume of the mouse ovum; and, second, beginning at blastocyst formation, late on day 3, the rabbit embryo increases very rapidly in mass. During the later period the rabbit blastocyst cannot easily be compared to the mouse blastocyst. However, during the preblastocyst period of development, when the embryos can be easily compared, both the mouse and rabbit embryo oxidize pyruvate and lactate to a much greater extent than they oxidize glucose. In addition, for each of the substrates, the rabbit embryo oxidizes from 2 to 5 times as much as the mouse embryo during the first 3 days of development.

Although the mouse and rabbit blastocyst differ in their rate of preimplantation expansion, one method of comparing metabolism is on the basis of oxygen consumption. The oxygen consumption has been measured for the rabbit embryo by Fridhandler [9] and for the mouse embryo by Mills & Brinster [10]. Table 4 shows a comparison of CO_2 production and oxygen uptake for each developmental stage of both embryos. Although there are some minor differences between the species, the outstanding observation is the similarity between the species in the way their embryos obtain energy. Pyruvate oxidation is able to account for 50–100 % of

oxygen uptake, depending on the developmental stage, for both species, and glucose oxidation can account for less than 5 % of the oxygen uptake of the newly ovulated ovum of both the mouse and rabbit. In both species glucose oxidation gradually increases up to the time of implantation. Lactate oxidation resembles pyruvate oxidation in most respects, but lactate does not seem to be oxidized as readily as pyruvate by the embryos.

These similarities mentioned above are striking when one considers the differences in the morphology, the reported culture requirements [1,

Table 4. *Molar ratio of radioactive carbon dioxide production compared to oxygen uptake in the preimplantation mouse and rabbit embryo*

Stage of development	Glucose		Pyruvate		Lactate	
	Mouse	Rabbit	Mouse	Rabbit	Mouse	Rabbit
Unfertilized	0.02	—	1.04	—	0.45	—
Fertilized	0.10	0.03	0.99	0.51	0.47	0.39
Day						
2	0.18	0.22	0.90	0.50	0.41	0.83
3	0.25	0.37	0.85	0.59	0.53	0.61
4	0.48	0.21	0.66	0.83	0.62	0.73
5	0.62	0.56	0.66	0.86	0.63	0.28
6	—	0.51	—	1.03	—	0.40

Substrate utilization is from table 3.
Oxygen consumption for the mouse was taken from Mills & Brinster [10], and for the rabbit from Fridhandler [9].

8], and the lactate dehydrogenase content of the preimplantation embryos of the 2 species [2, 6]. From the information available at the present time, there appears to be a distinct possibility that the energy source requirements and the energy metabolism of the preimplantation stages of pregnancy, particularly during the first 2–3 days of development, of many mammalian species may be quite similar.

I thank Miss Mary Ryans for her excellent technical assistance.

Financial support for this work was from the National Institutes of Health, grant HD 03071, and Pennsylvania Department of Agriculture (ME-8).

REFERENCES

1. Austin, C R, The mammalian egg. Thomas, Springfield, Ill. (1961).
2. Brinster, R L, Biochim biophys acta 110 (1965) 439.
3. — J reprod fertil 10 (1965) 227.
4. — Exptl cell res 47 (1967) 271.
5. — Ibid. 47 (1967) 634.
6. — Biochim biophys acta 148 (1967) 298.
7. — Exptl cell res. 51 (1968) 330.
8. — The mammalian oviduct (ed E S E Hafez & R Blandau). University of Chicago Press, New York (1968).
9. Fridhandler, L, Exptl cell res 22 (1961) 303.
10. Mills, R M, Jr & Brinster, R L, Exptl cell res 47 (1967) 337.

Patterns of Nucleic Acid Synthesis in the Early Mouse Embryo

K. A. O. ELLEM AND R. B. L. GWATKIN

INTRODUCTION

The central role of DNA as the library of the genetic information of a species, and of RNA as its mediator and distributor, suggests that a study of nucleic acid synthesis during development may provide a framework for probing the various control mechanisms that must operate during ontogenesis (reviews: Davis, 1964; Ebert and Kaighn, 1966). Since adequate supplies of amphibian and echinoderm zygotes are easily obtained, much is already known about nucleic acid synthesis during early development in these groups. However, it has been difficult to produce adequate quantities of mammalian zygotes. This problem has now been met by the use of hormonally induced superovulation in the mouse, and the availability of media that permit *in vitro* development of mouse eggs to the blastocyst stage (Gwatkin, 1966a). A further process of attachment to the culture vessel wall, which resembles implantation, also occurs *in vitro* (Gwatkin, 1966b).

This paper presents an exploratory study of the rates of synthesis of the different species of nucleic acid in mouse embryos. This has been achieved by the use of methylated bovine serum albumin-kieselguhr (MAK) chromatography for a one-step separation and analysis of precursor incorporation into the known varieties of nucleic acid, a method that has previously proved useful in analyzing the nucleic acid synthesis in very limited amounts of material (Miettinen *et al.*, 1966). Stages from 2 cell to blastocyst were employed. The subsequent phase of attachment and outgrowth of the blastocysts on a substratum *in vitro* was also examined. The study has defined several

111

phases in which large changes in the synthesis of specific nucleic acids occur, and indicates the path for further study of their specific role in the control of early differentiation.

MATERIALS AND METHODS

Embryos. These were obtained from Swiss mice, 6–8 weeks old, after their superovulation with gonadotropins. The techniques have been described elsewhere (Gwatkin, 1966c). Two-cell and 8-cell stages were taken directly from the oviduct. Morulae and blastocysts were cultured from the 2-cell stage in pyruvate-lactate medium (Brinster, 1965). Blastocysts were allowed to grow out on the bottom of a 60-mm plastic petri dish in 2 ml of Eagle's basal medium with 5% fetal calf serum (Gwatkin, 1966b).

Cell number. The mean number of cells in the mouse morulae, blastocysts, and blastocyst-outgrowths was measured by dissolving the cytoplasm with 1% sodium citrate. The free nuclei were then fixed with acetic alcohol, spread on a slide by air drying, and counted after staining with Giemsa. The procedure is a modification of an air-drying method for mouse embryo chromosome preparation (Tarkowski, 1966). The cells were counted in 10 embryos, and the standard error of the mean was calculated

Isotope incorporation. A known number of embryos of the appropriate stage was incubated at $37°C$ in 1 ml of pyruvate-lactate medium (Brinster, 1965) in a capped plastic tube. For blastocyst outgrowths, plastic petri dishes (60 mm in diameter) were used instead of the tubes and were incubated in an atmosphere of approximately 5% CO_2 and 95% air. At the beginning of the period of incubation, $50\mu C$ of uridine-^{3}H (5C/mmole, Nuclear Chicago) and 10 μC of thymidine-^{14}C (37.9 mC/mmole, Nuclear Chicago) was added. The incubation was performed routinely for 5 hours, with frequent manual agitation. At the end of the incubation period the embryos were collected on a 5 μ pore size membrane filter and the incubation medium saved for determination of the isotope concentration. The embryos were washed with 10 ml of culture medium, containing 2×10^6 L cells. The medium reduced the level of unused isotope, and the L cells provided carrier nucleic acids to guard against shear degradation of DNA (Hershey and Burgi, 1960) as well as to provide coprecipitants in processing and optical density markers in the subsequent analysis. The membrane was then immediately immersed in 5 ml of a solution of sodium dodecyl sulfate (SDS), and, after rapid shaking, the lysate was deproteinized with phenol as previously described (Ellem, 1966). The aqueous phase was removed as completely as possible and the nucleic acids were finally precipitated with 4 volumes of ethanol.

Nucleic acid analysis. After they had stood at $-20°C$ for at least 24 hours, the nucleic acids were recovered from the ethanolic fluid by filtration on membrane filters of 0.45 μ pore size. The membranes were washed with a solution of 2 volumes of ethanol and 1 volume of 0.3 M NaCl in 0.05 M Tris/HCl buffer pH 6.7 (0.3 M TBS). The nucleic acids were dissolved in 10 ml of 0.3 M TBS with shaking. The optical density of the solution was read at 260 mμ and the entire sample was applied to a column of methylated bovine serum albumin-coated kieselguhr. Chromatography was performed under the same conditions as described previously (Ellem, 1966) except that the size of the column was reduced to 0.5 $\times$ 8 cm and the total volume of the eluting fluids was 75 ml. A linear concentration gradient from 0.3 to 1.6 M TBS was used at 35°C, and was followed by an SDS solution at 35°C, and then at 80°C to elute the tenaciously bound DNA-like RNA (TD-RNA) (Ellem and Sheridan, 1964; Ellem, 1966). The eluate was scanned for ultraviolet-absorbing material, and 32-drop fractions were collected. Carrier yeast RNA was added to each tube; the nucleic acids precipitated and were collected on membrane filters, dissolved in NCS solubilizer (Nuclear Chicago), and counted in a Nuclear Chicago liquid scintillation spectrometer using a toluene dilution of Liquifluor, as described previously (Ellem, 1967). Quench correction was based on external standardization with the previously observed safeguards. Computation of the absolute disintegrations of ^{3}H and ^{14}C, counted simultaneously in the samples was performed with the aid of an IBM 1401 computer.

RESULTS

MAK Chromatography of Embryonic Nucleic Acids

Several batches of up to 600 two-cell eggs were processed, but too few counts were obtained after chromatography to provide reliable evidence of incorporation at this stage. However, the later stages studied had adequate incorporation. Figure 1 shows typical elution profiles of the total labeled nucleic acid fractions extracted from embryos after 5 hours of isotopic incorporation from the other four stages

113

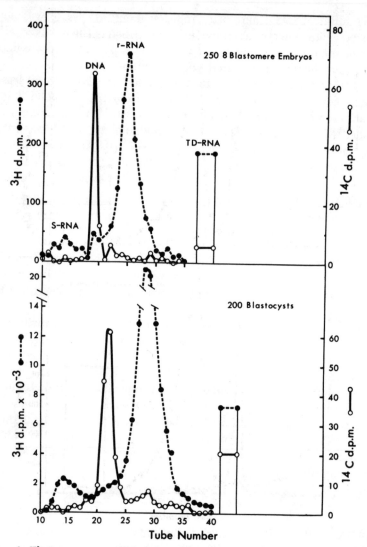

Fig. 1. Elution patterns of labeled nucleic acids from the early stages of mouse embryos. A MAK column was used and elution was accomplished by a linear gradient of sodium chloride from 0.3 M to 1.6 M as TBS. ^{3}H was supplied as uridine-^{3}H to label RNA and ^{14}C as thymidine-^{14}C to label DNA. TD-RNA is the DNA-like RNA eluted by SDS after completion of the salt gradient elution.

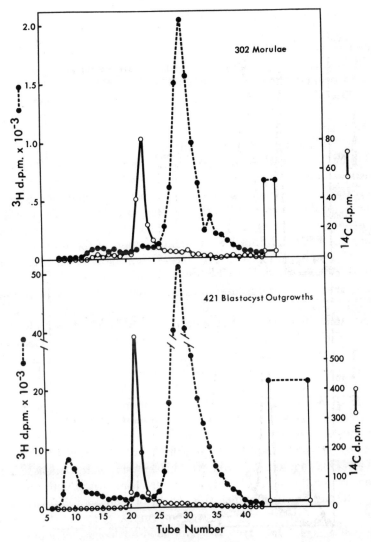

FIG. 1. (Continued).

studied. It can be seen that all these stages exhibited qualitatively the same elution pattern. The peaks of radioactivity corresponded to the appropriate nucleic acid peaks of the unlabeled carrier L cells inscribed by the recorder, but not shown in the figure. Uridine-^{3}H was incorporated into each major recognized RNA fraction, eluting in turn as sRNA, rRNA, and TD-RNA. The material eluting before DNA is designated sRNA. It includes tRNA, and 5sRNA (Galibert et al., 1967). The differences in the elution patterns of this material need further study to evaluate their significance. The TD-RNA contains the bulk of the DNA-like RNA of the cell, which is bound tenaciously by the basic protein of column (Ellem and Sheridan, 1964; Ellem, 1966; Lingrel, 1967; Ewing and Cherry, 1967). The DNA peak, defined by the selective incorporation of thymidine-^{14}C was typically abrupt in its elution. The overall elution pattern of the nucleic acids in the diagrams resembles that of other mammalian cells (e.g., Philipson, 1961; Ellem, 1966). There was a small amount of ^{3}H-incorporation beneath the DNA peak, which may be due in part to tailing of sRNA and in part to incorporation of the uridine-^{3}II as deoxycytidylate, into DNA (Comings, 1966). It represents a small fraction of the total labeling, and has not been further characterized. It will be referred to as D-H-UR in the results.

More than 90% of the isotope present in the TD-RNA of HeLa cells labeled for 5 hours or less has a DNA-like RNA composition, is rapidly labeled, and sediments in a pattern closely resembling polysomal mRNA (Ellem, 1966). Also, the synthesis of TD-RNA and DNA-like RNA are relatively unaffected by concentrations of actinomycin D that cause gross inhibition of rRNA synthesis (e.g., Perry, 1962; Perry et al., 1964; Clark and Ellem, 1966; Ellem, 1967). In order to verify that the RNA eluting in the TD-RNA fraction was relatively uncontaminated with rRNA, and was thus presumably DNA-like RNA with characteristics resembling mRNA of other mammalian cells, the resistance of its synthesis to actinomycin D was compared to that of rRNA in blastocysts. Accordingly, blastocysts were labeled with uridine-^{3}H and thymidine-^{14}C for 1 hour, for comparison with previous work with HeLa cells in which this length of incorporation was used, in the presence or absence of actinomycin D. Since Mintz (1964) found that 10^{-7} M actinomycin D suppressed nucleolar development in 4-cell mouse embryos, and also abolished nucleolar RNA synthesis (rRNA), without materially diminishing extranucleolar RNA synthesis (mainly DNA-like RNA), this concentration was used. The data in Fig. 2 and Table 1 show gross inhibition of rRNA and sRNA synthesis with virtually no effect on the synthesis of TD-RNA, and little effect on that of DNA. Thus, the response of high molecular weight RNA

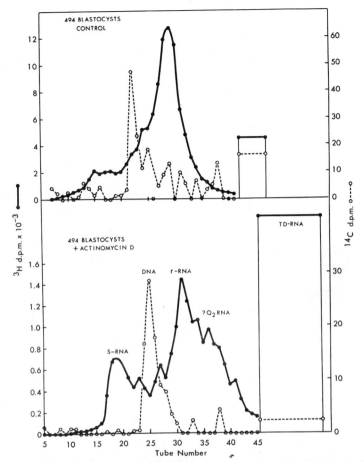

Fig. 2. Effects of $10^{-7}\,M$ actinomycin D on the 1 hour labeling pattern of RNA in mouse blastocysts. Labeling conditions described in text. Note that different scales are used for the control and the treated groups. The gross inhibition of sRNA and of rRNA synthesis is evident, while the synthesis of the DNA-like RNA (TD-RNA) is relatively unaffected. Inhibition of rRNA reveals the presence of a component that may be analogous to Q2-RNA in other cells (see text).

synthesis to actinomycin, as well as its chromatographic properties was similar in the embryonic material to that of other cells. It is, therefore, considered to be DNA-like RNA. Any slight contamination of the TD-RNA fraction by rRNA (usually no more than 5–10% of the isotope present in the rRNA fraction when ^{32}P was used) (Ellem, 1966), will

TABLE 1

Selective Effects of a Low Dose (10^{-7} M) of Actinomycin
on the Synthesis of MAK Separated Nucleic Acids
from Mouse Blastocysts

Nucleic acid	Experiment 1			Experiment 2		
	370[a] Control	370+ actinomycin	Percent inhibition	494 Control	494+ actinomycin	Percent inhibition
sRNA	16,126[b]	4,875	69.8	16,628	2,862	82.8
D-H-UR[d]	10,391	3,183	69.4	19,682	2,937	84.9
rRNA	106,522	31,228	70.7	73,757	12,319	83.3
TD-RNA	17,820	17,561	1.5	22,694	24,641	−8.3
Total	150,859	56,847	62.3	126,117	41,679	76.9
DNA	123.0[c]	96.5	21.5	104.8	81.3	22.4

[a] Number of blastocysts in sample.

[b] Total dpm. ^{3}H incorporated into fraction during 1 hour of exposure to 50 μC uridine-^{3}H per milliliter at 37°C.

[c] Total dpm. ^{14}C incorporated into DNA peak during 1 hour of exposure to 10 μC thymidine-^{14}C per milliliter at 37°C.

[d] Incorporated ^{3}H from uridine-^{3}H eluting with the DNA peak, in material which has not yet been defined (see text).

tend to reduce any differences that might be observed in the behavior of rRNA and DNA-like RNA. Such differences when observed, will thus be all the more significant.

Quantitative Changes in Precursor Incorporation into Nucleic Acids during Development

The overall rates of precursor incorporation into nucleic acid which occur at each stage were calculated as the mean of the total amount of each isotope incorporated in two separate experiments for each stage under consideration. Table 2 contains the data, obtained as the sum of the individual fractions isolated by MAK chromatography. As might be anticipated, incorporation into total RNA increased dramatically in the whole embryo from the 8-cell stage to outgrowth of the blastocyst. More meaningful values are obtained when these results are expressed in relation to the number of cells present at each stage. It can be seen that there was a major step up in the rate of incorporation into RNA per cell following the transition from the 8-cell to the morula (Table 2). There was little change in total RNA incorporation per cell from the morula to the blastocyst. However, after outgrowth

TABLE 2

Total Incorporation of Uridine-³H and Thymidine-¹⁴C into Different Stages of Developing Embryos

Developmental stage	8-Cell	Morula (21 ± 1)[b]	Blastocyst (107 ± 4)	Blastocyst outgrowth (117 ± 6)
Whole Embryo				
RNA	1300 ± 120[a]	22,300 ± 1500	132,100 ± 4,900	388,000 ± 24,000
DNA	240 ± 40	900 ± 270	430 ± 110	3,190 ± 1,050
DNA/RNA	0.18	0.044	0.0032	0.0082
Per Cell				
RNA	163 ± 15	1,060 ± 70	1,230 ± 50	3,320 ± 200
	30 ± 5	47 ± 13	4 ± 1	27 ± 9

[a] Values are expressed as dpm. ³H or ¹⁴C incorporated by 100 embryos/10⁸ dpm precursor per milliliter of medium in 5 hours at 37°C. They represent the mean of 2 separate analyses ± the range of the duplicates.

[b] Numbers in parentheses represent the number of cells ± standard error of the mean.

of the blastocysts there was a further increase in the rate of precursor incorporation into RNA, amounting to 3 times that of the blastocysts before outgrowth.

The average DNA synthesis per cell was most rapid in the morula and only a little less so in the 8-cell embryo. After establishment of the blastocyst, DNA synthesis was reduced by about 90%. After the blastocyst grew out on the wall of the culture vessel, DNA synthesis resumed and increased to approximately the same rate as in the 8-cell stage.

Change among Different Types of Nucleic Acid

To specify the types of RNA involved in the variations of synthesis which were detected at different stages, the behavior of the individual RNA fractions in relation to one another was examined. Table 3 shows the data for the distribution of ^{3}H, incorporated into the DNA-like RNA. The relative synthesis of the DNA-like RNA fraction was less

TABLE 3

PERCENTAGE DISTRIBUTION OF ISOTOPE AMONG NUCLEIC ACIDS
AFTER 5 HOURS' EXPOSURE TO ^{3}H-URIDINE

| Nucleic acid | Embryonic stage | | | |
	8-Cell	Morula	Blastocyst	Blastocyst outgrowths
sRNA	10.2 ± 1.1^a	5.9 ± 0.3	8.2 ± 0.8	10.4 ± 1.9
D-H-UR[b]	8.1 ± 3.7	4.0 ± 0.3	6.5 ± 1.5	3.0 ± 1.1
rRNA	63.9 ± 2.2	82.0 ± 3.6	68.7 ± 1.2	62.3 ± 6.2
TD-RNA	17.9 ± 7.0	8.2 ± 3.0	16.7 ± 1.8	24.3 ± 9.1

[a] Values are the mean of two analyses ± range of duplicates.
[b] Incorporated ^{3}H from uridine-^{3}H eluting with DNA peak.

than had previously been found in cell cultures grown in vitro (Ellem, 1966). Therefore, a direct comparison was made, after 1 hour of isotope incorporation, between blastocysts, blastocyst outgrowths, and a strain of diploid fibroblasts at a stage of growth close to forming a monolayer. The results in Table 4 verify that the preimplantation stages synthesize relatively less DNA-like RNA than the blastocysts after outgrowth, and also that the distribution pattern of incorporation after the blastocysts attach to a surface resembles closely that of monolayer cultures of diploid cells.

To express the relative rates of incorporation into the nucleic acid

TABLE 4

COMPARISON OF PERCENTAGE DISTRIBUTION OF URIDINE-^{3}H AFTER 1 HOUR
OF EXPOSURE TO URIDINE-^{3}H BETWEEN BLASTOCYST
AND DIPLOID CELLS IN VITRO

Nucleic acid	Blastocysts	Blastocyst outgrowths	WI38[b]
sRNA	11.9 ± 1.2[a]	3.1 ± 0.2	3.2 ± 0.3
D-H-UR[c]	11.3 ± 4.4	1.9 ± 0.4	1.9 ± 0.1
rRNA	61.9 ± 8.7	49.9 ± 4.2	44.9 ± 1.7
TD-RNA	14.9 ± 3.1	45.2 ± 4.8	50.1 ± 2.2

[a] Values are the mean of two analyses ± range of duplicates.

[b] Percent distribution of uridine-^{3}H among fractions of nucleic acids from mono-layers of human diploid (WI38) cells.

[c] Incorporated ^{3}H eluting with the DNA peak.

fraction at each stage, the isotope incorporation into each fraction was calculated on a per cell basis. For the purpose of comparison, each was then expressed relative to the incorporation rate of 8-cell embryos, which were assigned the value of 1.00. The rate of incorporation into rRNA showed an abrupt increase at the morula stage, to 8 times that of the 8-cell stage, which was maintained during blastulation. On the other hand, sRNA and DNA-like RNA (TD-RNA) showed a gradually increasing rate of incorporation. The overall rate of incorporation of

TABLE 5

RELATIVE RATES OF PRECURSOR INCORPORATION INTO INDIVIDUAL
NUCLEIC ACID FRACTIONS PER CELL DURING DEVELOPMENT

Nucleic acid	Morula	Blastocyst	Blastocyst outgrowths
sRNA	3.77[a]	6.08	20.8
D-H-UR[b]	3.21	6.06	7.57
rRNA	8.34	8.11	19.9
TD-RNA	2.98	7.03	27.7
Total	6.50	7.54	20.4
DNA[c]	1.57	0.13	0.89

[a] RNA figures calculated from mean incorporation of uridine-^{3}H per fraction per cell following 5 hours' isotope incorporation in 2 separate experiments for each embryonic stage. Values compared to 8-cell stage as 1.00.

[b] Figures based on ^{3}H chromatographing beneath the DNA peak as defined by thymidine-^{14}C incorporation.

[c] DNA figures calculated from mean incorporation of ^{14}C-thymidine chromatographing in the DNA peak per cell.

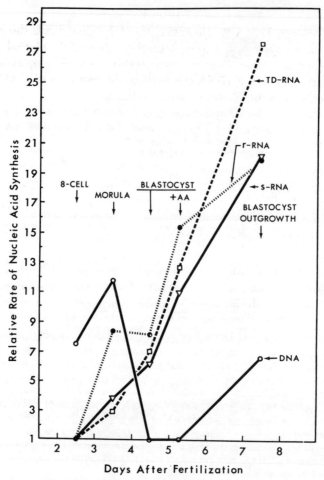

Fig. 3. Relative rates of incorporation of precursor into each nucleic acid species n the embryos in relation to the time elapsed after fertilization. The rates of incorporation into RNA are calculated on a per cell basis relative to the 8-cell stage, which is arbitrarily assigned a value of 1.0. The DNA figures, also calculated on per cell basis, are normalized to the rate in blastocysts, rather than to the 8-cell :age.

H-uridine, since the rRNA contained the bulk of the label, exhibited marked increase in the morula with little change up to the blastocyst. Comparison of the rates of incorporation into nucleic acids of the lastocyst before and after outgrowth showed an acceleration in all moieties except D-H-UR. However, the DNA-like RNA showed the largest relative increase. Figure 3 displays these data plotted against the approximate time elapsed since fertilization. It emphasizes the selective stimulation of rRNA synthesis in the morula and of DNA-like RNA synthesis in the blastocyst outgrowths.

The ability of the blastocyst to grow out *in vitro* is dependent on several amino acids and one or more factors supplied by serum

TABLE 6

EFFECTS OF ARGININE AND LEUCINE ON PRECURSOR INCORPORATION
INTO BLASTOCYST NUCLEIC ACIDS

Nucleic acid	Experiment 1[a]			Experiment 2[b] Dual Isotope Method (% increase)
	133 Blastocysts without AA	133 Blastocysts with AA	Increase as % initial value	
sRNA	6,436	12,762	198	166
D-H-UR[c]	3,586	7,993	223	144
rRNA	48,470	97,810	202	158
TD-RNA	13,280	19,517	147	175
Total	71,772	138,082	192	171
DNA[d]	47.3	51.0	108	—

[a] Total incorporation of uridine-^{3}H and thymidine-^{14}C as dpm in 5 hours, as in Methods.

[b] Estimated by the use of the dual label method as outlined in the text. The experiment used 2 pairs of blastocyst cultures, one of each pair having been supplied with 10^{-4} M arginine and 2×10^{-4} M leucine. Pairs were labeled for 5 hours in the presence of either cytidine-^{14}C (10 μC/ml; 256 mC/mmole) or cytidine-^{3}H (50 μC/ml; 1830 mC/mmole). the amino acid-stimulated culture receiving cytidine-^{14}C in one pair and cytidine-^{3}H in the other. The control cultures lacking arginine and leucine were labeled with the precursor containing the other isotope. At the end of incubation the 2 cultures of a pair were collected on the one membrane and processed together as outlined in text.

[c] D-H-UR represents the incorporated isotope eluting with DNA.

[d] DNA as total incorporation of thymidine-^{14}C dpm/5 hours eluting in the DNA peak.

(Gwatkin, 1966b). It was, thus, of interest to observe the effect of the essential amino acids on nucleic acid synthesis in blastocysts supplied in medium containing the other factors necessary for outgrowth. In Table 6, the incorporation into each nucleic acid is shown, in replicate samples of blastocysts, in the presence and absence of arginine and leucine: both shown to be essential for outgrowth (Gwatkin, 1966b). It is clear that the incorporation into all RNA types was stimulated when these amino acids were present. The DNA-like RNA showed a little less stimulation than the others. At this time there was no demonstrable effect on DNA synthesis.

To confirm these results the experiment was repeated using another experimental design. The technique was that previously described for the elimination of column to column variation, and permits the simultaneous extraction, purification and chromatography of the nucleic acids from the control and experimental cells (Ellem, 1967). The method involves simultaneous labeling of the two cultures being compared, one with ^{14}C-labeled precursor, the other with the same precursor labeled with ^{3}H. At the end of the incubation the samples are mixed and processed together. A second set of cultures is handled similarly except that the isotopes are reversed between control and experimental cells. Calculations using the ^{3}H/^{14}C ratios of each fraction yield the relative rates of precursor incorporation of the experimental cells as a percentage of the control rate. The results of this experiment are listed in Table 6 (experiment 2) and agree fairly well with those based on simple quantitation. It is clear that the addition of arginine and leucine led to a general stimulation of incorporation into RNA which, by 19 hours had no marked selectivity for any particular moiety. Incorporation as a whole increased to 171% of the unstimulated value.

DISCUSSION

This study has measured the amount of incorporation of isotope from a labeled nucleoside precursor into a nucleic acid species in a 5-hour incubation time. In studies of macromolecular synthesis the assumption is customarily made, but less often stated, that the isotopic incorporation is a valid measure of synthesis. Its validity depends on the precursor nucleoside triphosphate pools reaching the same specific activity with similar kinetics in the different cells being compared, so that the amount of isotope incorporated into nucleic acid can be equated with the total amount of precursor (endogenous and exogenous) used in its synthesis. For short labeling times alterations in the rate at which the cell will take up precursor, and alterations in the size of the intracellular pools could affect the specific activity of the nucleoside triphosphates. In this study it has not been experimentally feasible to monitor the specific activity of the pools. In this discussion, the assumption will be made that precursor pool effects are small during the relatively long incubation with precursor (5 hours), and that differences in pool specific activities are not responsible for the observed differences in rates of incorporation into nucleic acid (termed synthesis) between different embryonic stages. However, until it is feasible to monitor the specific activities of the immediate nucleoside triphosphate precursors, the possible influence of this factor on the magnitude of the differences observed must be kept in mind.

Where differential effects are observed between different fractions of RNA, this is most unlikely to be the consequence of pool changes. In the following discussion the rates of synthesis that have been determined in this study are correlated with known biological events and independent analyses of total RNA content of the different embryonic stages, obtained from Reamer (1963).

The principal findings of this study are: (1) the extremely low rate of nucleic acid synthesis in the 2-cell embryo, and the low overall rate of RNA synthesis at the 8-cell stage; (2) the abrupt acceleration of the synthesis of rRNA in the morula to a level which then remains constant up to the end of the blastocyst stage, followed by a further elevation in the rate of precursor incorporation into rRNA following blastocyst outgrowth; (3) the gradual steady increase in the rate of synthesis of sRNA, D-H-UR, and DNA-like RNA up to the end of the blastocyst stage, followed by a further increase in sRNA synthesis and a much larger increase in DNA-like RNA synthesis after outgrowth; (4) the shutdown of DNA synthesis after blastocyst formation, and the resumption of DNA synthesis after blastocyst outgrowth. These results will be discussed in detail below.

(1 and 2) The mammalian ovum contains approximately 100 times the complement of ribosomal RNA present in adult cells (Reamer, 1963). Analysis of the first 5 cell doublings of mouse embryos revealed a steady fall in the RNA content of each cell until a level of 50.4 pg/cell was reached at the 16-blastomere stage (Reamer, 1963). Thus, the individual cells of the morula (21-cell stage) have an RNA content which is similar to that of an adult cell. In the absence of rRNA synthesis, further cell division would deplete the cell RNA content below optimal levels. The present observation that the onset of rapid rRNA synthesis occurred between the 8 cell and morula stages and was maintained thereafter, suggests that it is in fact necessary to replenish the cell reserves of rRNA at this stage. Monesi and Salfi (1967) have also observed large changes in uridine-^{3}H incorporation into RNA of mouse morulae which they also interpret as increased RNA synthesis. The detection of some rRNA synthesis in the first few blastomeres cor-

relates with previous observations that mammalian eggs are unique in possessing nucleoli in the early cleavage nuclei (e.g., Mintz, 1964, 1965). As is now well documented (Perry, 1962; Clark *et al.*, 1966) the nucleolus is the organelle concerned with the synthesis of rRNA. It is of interest to contrast the later onset of rRNA synthesis in the late blastula of amphibian eggs (Nemer, 1963; Brown and Littna, 1965). These eggs are very much larger than mammalian eggs and contain a much greater complement of rRNA (Brown, 1965). Ribosomal RNA synthesis begins in them at a stage which is composed of 150 times as many cells (the late amphibian blastula has 15,000 cells; Brown, 1965) as their mammalian counterpart.

In the present studies the fact that the rate of rRNA synthesis at the 8-cell stage was only 12% of that of the morula cannot be attributed solely to a low rate of uptake of precursor by the 8-cell embryos, or to a large pyrimidine pool in them, since the difference between the rates of synthesis of sRNA and TD-RNA at the two stages is very much less, and these are probably synthesized from the same nucleotide pool as the rRNA. It is clear that the interval between the 8-cell stage and morula represents a critical stage in the activation of the ribosomal cistrons during development, and will be worthy of further study to determine the initiating mechanism.

(3) The identification of TD-RNA with the bulk of the DNA-like RNA of the embryos is based on its similarities to the same moiety in other mammalian cells with respect to chromatographic properties and the selective resistance of its synthesis to actinomycin D. In HeLa cells, L cells and human diploid cells TD-RNA has the composition, rapidity of labeling, and sedimentation characteristics of mRNA (Ellem, 1966, 1967; Rhode and Ellem, 1968). Similar material has been found in other systems (Lingrel, 1967; Ewing and Cherry, 1967).

The steady increase in the rate of synthesis of DNA-like RNA (TD-RNA) might be interpreted to suggest a gradual increase in the number of genes being transcribed in the genome with the increasing demands for synthetic diversity, which accompany differentiation. The low rate of synthesis of TD-RNA relative to rRNA noted in the comparison with blastocyst outgrowths, embryonic fibroblasts and other cell types in cell culture may imply the presence of long-lived mRNA or possibly preprogrammed polyribosomes in the early stages of cleavage as have been found in amphibian and echinoderm eggs (e.g., Spirin, 1966). However, the assessment of this fraction awaits further understanding of the heterogeneity, function, and stability of the

DNA-like RNA. While a gradual increase in the rate of isotope incorporation into sRNA together with some changes in the elution pattern occurred as the embryo developed, their significance awaits characterization of the moieties concerned.

The 2- to 4-fold increase in the rate of incorporation of precursor into the various RNA fractions following outgrowth of the blastocyst may either represent an alteration in the handling of precursor (see above) or an overall activation in the synthesis of all RNA species. The fact that there is little change in the "D-H-UR" does not necessarily exclude the possibility of pool effects. Apart from the question of absolute change in rate of RNA synthesis, it is clear that there is a change in pattern following outgrowth, so that the TD-RNA fraction receives a greater amount of the precursor than at earlier stages. The pattern at outgrowth resembles that of tissue culture cells. Clearly the dramatic changes in precursor incorporation as a result of supplying the required amino acids and the ensuing steps of attachment and outgrowth demand further study as possible manifestations of induced genomic switches.

(4) The virtual cessation of DNA synthesis in the late blastocyst correlates well with the static condition at this stage in the absence of amino acids (Gwatkin, 1966a,b). After exposure to these amino acids the general increase in RNA metabolism affecting all moieties possibly reflects reactivation of the genome for outgrowth and changes within the trophoblast cells. These changes are enlargement of the nuclei and a branching and extrusion of the nucleoli (Gwatkin, 1966b). Nuclear enlargement may represent the opening-up of condensed chromatin as the genome becomes functional. Harris (1965) has noted such nuclear expansion when rat lymphocyte or chicken erythrocyte nuclei are induced to synthesize DNA and RNA in response to fusion with cultured human tumor cells. The resumption of DNA synthesis correlates with the observed mitosis following attachment (Gwatkin and Meckley, 1966). The present exploratory work has described only a late phase (after 19 hours) of this amino acid stimulation. Further work will be directed toward determining the more immediate responses.

SUMMARY

Nucleic acid synthesis was examined in the early mouse embryo during cleavage, blastulation, and outgrowth of the blastocyst on an artifical substratum. Rates of synthesis were inferred from the rate of incorporation of isotopically labeled precursors into DNA, sRNA, rRNA, and DNA-like RNA, separated by MAK chromatography. The following conclusions emerged: (1) Nucleic acid synthesis in the 2-blastomere egg was undetectable by the methods used. (2) Incorporation into all nucleic acid fractions was detectable at the 8-cell stage. (3) Measured on a per cell basis, there was abrupt acceleration of the precursor incorporation into rRNA in the morula to a level that was maintained up to the blastocyst stage. Further elevation of incorporation accompanied *in vitro* attachment and outgrowth of the blastocyst. (4) sRNA and DNA-like RNA showed a gradual steady increase in the rate of incorporation per cell up to the late blastocyst stage. Following blastocyst outgrowth there was a disproportionately great increase in the synthesis of DNA-like RNA. (5) The incorporation of thymidine-^{14}C into DNA virtually ceased in the late blastocyst; but resumed on outgrowth. (6) The incorporation into nucleic acids rose 19 hours after providing all the nutritional factors previously found to be necessary for blastocyst outgrowth. (7) The DNA-like RNA was synthesized at a low rate relative to rRNA when the early cleavage stages were compared with blastocyst outgrowths, or with fibroblasts and other cell types in cell culture. This may imply that m-RNA is long lived in the early stages of cleavage.

The authors wish to thank Mr. D. T. Williams and Miss Agnes T. Masse for skilled technical assistance. Mr. R. A. Cohen of the Jefferson Medical College and Medical Center Management Services generously provided computer facilities, and Mr. K. Brossoie is to be thanked for writing the program. This work was supported by USPHS Grants 2RO1 CA-05402-08 and 5TO1 GM-00813-06.

REFERENCES

Brinster, R. L. (1965). Studies on the development of mouse embryos *in vitro*. IV. Interaction of energy sources. *J. Reprod. Fertility* 10, 227–240.

Brown, D. D. (1965). RNA synthesis during early development. In "Developmental and Metabolic Control Mechanisms and Neoplasia," pp. 219–234. Williams & Wilkins, Baltimore, Maryland.

Brown, D. D., and Littna, E. (1965). RNA synthesis during the development of *Xenopus laevis*, the South African clawed toad. *J. Mol. Biol.* 8, 669–687.

Clark, A. M., and Ellem, K. A. O. (1966). A correlated morphological and functional study of the effects of actinomycin D on HeLa cells. II. The selective effects of low concentrations of the rapidly labeled types of RNA separated by column chromatography. *Ann. Med. Exptl. Biol. Fenniae* (*Helsinki*) 44, 100–108.

Clark, A. M., Love, R., Studzinski, G. P., and Ellem, K. A. O. (1966). A correlated morphological and functional study of the effects of actinomycin D on HeLa cells. I. Effects of the nucleolar and cytoplasmic ribonucleoproteins. *Exptl. Cell Res.* **45**, 106–119.

COMINGS, D. E. (1966). Incorporation of tritium of ^{3}H-5-uridine into DNA. *Exptl. Cell Res.* **41**, 677–681.

DAVIS, B. D. (1964). Theoretical mechanisms of differentiation. *Medicine* **43**, 639–649.

EBERT, J. D., and KAIGHN, M. E. (1966). The keys to change: factors regulating differentiation. *In* "Major Problems in Developmental Biology" (M. Locke, ed.), pp. 29–84. Academic Press, New York.

ELLEM, K. A. O. (1966). Some properties of the DNA-like RNA of mammalian cells isolated by chromatography on columns of methylated bovine serum albumin. *J. Mol. Biol.* **20**, 283–305.

ELLEM, K. A. O. (1967). A dual label technique for comparing the rates of synthesis of MAK separated nucleic acid fractions from cells in different states of activity. *Biochim. Biophys. Acta* **149**, 74–87.

ELLEM, K. A. O., and SHERIDAN, J. W. (1964). Tenacious binding of the DNA-like RNA of metazoan cells to columns of methylated serum albumin. *Biochem. Biophys. Res. Commun.* **16**, 505–510.

EWING, E. E., and CHERRY, J. H. (1967). Base composition and column chromatography studies of ribonucleic acid differentially extracted from pea roots with sodium lauryl sulphate or p-amino salicylate. *Phytochemistry* **6**, 1319–1328.

GALIBERT, F., LELONG, J. C., LARSEN, C. J., and BOIRON, M. (1967). Position of 5s-RNA among cellular ribonucleic acids. *Biochim. Biophys. Acta* **142**, 89–98.

GWATKIN, R. B. L. (1966a). Defined media and development of mammalian eggs *in vitro. Ann. N. Y. Acad. Sci.* **139**, 79–90

GWATKIN, R. B. L. (1966b). Amino acid requirements for attachment and outgrowth of the mouse blastocyst *in vitro. J. Cell Physiol.* **68**, 335–343.

GWATKIN, R. B. L. (1966c). Effect of viruses on early mammalian development. III. Further studies concerning the interaction of Mengo encephalitis virus with mouse ova. *Fertility Sterility* **17**, 411–420.

GWATKIN, R. B. L., and MECKLEY, D. E. (1966). Chromosomes of the mouse blastocyst following its attachment and outgrowth *in vitro. Ann. Med. Exptl. Biol. Fenniae (Helsinki)* **44**, 125–127.

HARRIS, H. (1963). Nuclear ribonucleic acid. *Progr. Nucleic Acid Res.* **2**, 19–59.

HARRIS, H. (1965). Behaviour of differentiated nuclei in heterokaryons of animal cells from different species. *Nature* **206**, 583–588.

HERSHEY, A. D., and BURGI, E. (1960). Molecular homogeneity of the deoxyribonucleic acid of phage T2. *J. Mol. Biol.* **2**, 143–152.

LINGREL, J. B. (1967). Studies on the rapidly labeled RNA of rabbit bone marrow cells. *Biochim. Biophys. Acta* **142**, 75–88.

MIETTINEN, H., ELLEM, K. A. O., and SAXÉN, L. (1966). Studies on kidney tubulogenesis. VII. The response of RNA synthesis of mouse metanephrogenic mesenchyme to an inductive stimulus. *Ann. Med. Exptl. Biol. Fenniae (Helsinki)* **44**, 109–116.

MINTZ, B. (1964). Synthetic processes and early development in the mammalian egg. *J. Exptl. Zool.* **157**, 85–100.

MINTZ, B. (1965). Nucleic acid and protein synthesis in the developing mouse embryo. *In* "Preimplantation Stages of Pregnancy" (G. E. W. Wolstenholme and M. O'Conner, eds.), pp. 145–155. Little, Brown, Boston, Massachusetts.

MONESI, V., and SALFI, V. (1967). Macromolecular synthesis during early development in the mouse embryo. *Exptl. Cell Res.* 46, 632–635.

NEMER, M. (1963). Old and new RNA in the embryogenesis of the purple sea urchin. *Proc. Natl. Acad. Sci. U. S.* 50, 230–235.

PERRY, R. P. (1962). The cellular sites of synthesis of ribosomal and 4s RNA. *Proc. Natl. Acad. Sci. U. S.* 48, 2179–2186.

PERRY, R. P., SRINIVASAN, P. R., and KELLEY, D. B. (1964). Hybridization of rapidly labeled nuclear ribonucleic acids. *Science* 145, 504–507.

PHILIPSON, L. (1961). Chromatographic separation, and characteristics of nucleic acids from HeLa cells. *J. Gen. Physiol.* 44, 899–910.

REAMER, G. R. (1963). The quantity and distribution of nucleic acids in the early cleavage stages of the mouse embryo. Ph. D. Thesis, Boston University.

RHODE, S. L., and ELLEM, K. A. O. (1968). The control of nucleic acid synthesis during contact inhibition of human embryonic fibroblasts. *Exptl. Cell Res.* in press.

SPIRIN, A. S. (1966). On "masked forms" of messenger RNA in early embryogenesis and in other differentiating systems. *In* "Current Topics in Developmental Biology" (A. A. Moscona and A. Monroy, eds.), Vol. 1, pp. 1–38. Academic Press, New York.

TARKOWSKI, A. K. (1966). An air-drying method for chromosome preparations from mouse eggs. *Cytogenetics* 5, 394–400.

130

Effects of Actinomycin D and Cycloheximide on RNA and Protein Synthesis in Cleavage Stage Mouse Embryos

by
RICHARD J. TASCA
NINA HILLMAN

THERE have been several reports on the effects of actinomycin D on the morphological development of cleavage stage mouse embryos[1-4]. These studies show that low concentrations of actinomycin D ($1–2 \times 10^{-4}$ µg/ml.) have no effect on the rate of cleavage or on blastocyst development. Intermediate concentrations (6×10^{-4} to 1×10^{-3} µg/ml.) do not interfere with cell division during cleavage but prevent blastocyst differentiation (expansion, elongation, hatching) when the antibiotic treatment begins at the late four cell or older stages. Cells of embryos treated with higher concentrations (> 0.08 µg/ml.) undergo no more than one additional mitotic division before development is arrested.

Autoradiographic and cytochemical studies have shown that intermediate concentrations of actinomycin D cause a reduction of nucleolar RNA synthesis, while higher concentrations reduce, or block, all nuclear RNA synthesis[2]. There is only a slight reduction of protein synthesis as a result of these treatments. The sensitivity of cleavage stage embryos to a protein synthesis inhibitor (puromycin) has been described[1]. These studies show that there is a correlation between the dosage of puromycin and the stage at which development is blocked. There have been, however, no detailed biochemical analyses to determine the effects of antibiotics on RNA and protein syntheses during early mouse development. The present study reports the effects of actinomycin D and cycloheximide on the rates of RNA and protein synthesis in two cell to morula (sixteen to thirty-two cells) stage mouse embryos.

For this study, large numbers of synchronously developing, two cell embryos were obtained from 10–12 week old superovulated[5] albino females which had been mated to albino males. The embryos were placed in mouse embryo culture medium[6] in which they developed from the two cell stage to the blastocyst (more than thirty-two cells) stage in approximately two days. The two cell embryos were allowed to develop to specific cleavage stages and were

131

then incubated in either ^{3}H-5-uridine (6 μCi/ml., 20–25 Ci/mmole, Schwartz) or in ^{14}C-leucine (0·6 μCi/ml., 170–200 mCi/mmole, Schwartz) fJr a 3 h period in the presence or absence of actinomycin D or cycloheximide. The embryonic stages treated were: late two cell (L2); late two cell–early four cell (L2E4); early four cell (E4); late four cell (L4); eight to sixteen cell; and late morula (LM, sixteen to thirty-two cells). After the 3 h incubation those embryos to be used for biochemical studies were counted, rinsed four times with culture medium, collected in 20 μl. of Earle's BSS, frozen in solid CO_2 and acetone and stored at − 70° C. The remaining embryos were washed, placed into unlabelled culture medium and allowed to continue development so that the effects of the drugs on development could be determined. Each experiment was repeated at least three times.

A modified Schmidt–Thannhauser[7] technique was used for extracting the embryos. After thawing the embryos, 25 μl. of cold distilled water was added, and the embryos were ruptured by four freeze–thawings. Cold 1·6 M perchloric acid (PCA) was added to obtain a final concentration of 0·3 M PCA. This treatment was followed by ribonuclease (0·2 per cent) digestion of the acid-insoluble precipitate and then hyamine hydroxide digestion of the residual ribonuclease resistant pellet. All centrifugations were performed at 13,000 r.p.m. for 20 min and all precipitates were washed twice. These steps provided the following three fractions: acid soluble; acid insoluble, ribonuclease sensitive (RNA fraction); acid insoluble, ribonuclease resistant, hyamine hydroxide soluble (protein fraction). The amount of label contained in each fraction was determined by liquid scintillation counting. The total of the counts of the acid soluble fraction (unincorporated precursor), RNA fraction and protein fraction accounts for all of the radioactive label which enters the embryos and is designated as ^{3}H-5-uridine uptake or ^{14}C-leucine uptake.

In initial experiments it was found that the ^{3}H-5-uridine uptake (in c.p.m./100 embryos) increased by three-fold between the L4 stage and eight to sixteen cell stage, and by four-fold between the eight to sixteen cell stage and morula stage (Fig. 3). For this reason, the rates of RNA and protein synthesis are here expressed as "percentage incorporation", or the total number of counts in the RNA or protein fraction/total uptake of precursor × 100. The data are expressed as percentage incorporation so that syntheses of different stages may be compared despite permeability differences which may be reflexions of changes in the endogenous precursor pool sizes (not yet determined in mouse embryos). Treating the data in this way, it was found that the rates of synthesis are characteristic for each stage, for the percentage incorporation does not fluctuate significantly when the uptake of the precursors is changed by incubating the embryos with different amounts of radioactivity: ^{3}H-5-uridine (1·5–25 μCi/ml.) or ^{14}C-leucine (0·3 to 0·6 μCi/ml.).

The rate of RNA synthesis increases progressively in cleavage stage mouse embryos from 8 per cent at the late two cell stage to 30 per cent at the morula stage (RNA controls, Fig. 1). The largest increase (9 per cent) occurs between the eight to sixteen cell stage and the morula stage. Recently, it was reported that high molecular weight RNA synthesis is detectable as early as the two cell stage, and ribosomal RNA (rRNA) synthesis at the four cell stage[8]. Moreover, rRNA synthesis has been

132

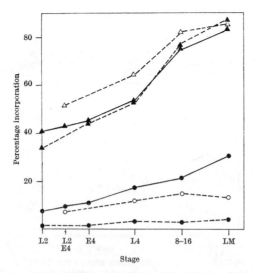

Fig. 1. Effects of actinomycin D on the rates of RNA and protein synthesis in cleavage stage mouse embryos. ^{14}C-leucine: ▲—▲, control; △ - - - △, +0·0008 μg/ml. actinomycin D; ▲ - - -▲, +0·1 μg/ml. actinomycin D. ^{3}H-5-uridine: ●—●, control; ○ - - - ○, +0·0008 μg/ml. actinomycin D; ● - - - ●, +0·1 μg/ml. actinomycin D.

shown to increase at the eight cell and morula stages[9]. The increases can be correlated with a progressive hypertrophy of the pars granulosa of the nucleoli at each successive developmental stage[10]. Granular nucleoli are first present at the L2 stage, suggesting that part of the RNA which is synthesized at this stage is rRNA or rRNA precursor molecules.

Evidence which supports the above findings, that rRNA is synthesized in early mouse embryos, is provided by actinomycin D experiments (Fig. 1). Actinomycin D (0·0008 μg/ml.) reduces the rate of RNA synthesis at all stages. The rate of synthesis is reduced slightly at the L2–E4 stage (approximately 2 per cent). This reduction becomes greater through the cleavage stages until the morula stage when the percentage incorporation is about 14 per cent (16 per cent reduction from the normal value). Because low concentrations of actinomycin D preferentially inhibit rRNA synthesis[11], it is probable that most, if not all, of the mouse embryo RNA synthesis which is inhibited by 0·0008 μg/ml. actinomycin D is rRNA. Although this concentration of antibiotic allows embryos, regardless of stage of treatment, to form blastocysts, treatment at the eight to sixteen cell stage and at the morula stage prevents blastocyst differentiation (present work and others)[3]. A higher drug concentration (0·1 μg/ml.), which inhibits cell division, severely inhibits RNA synthesis at all stages (Fig. 1).

When rates of protein synthesis in mouse embryos are measured (controls, Fig. 1), it can be seen that 41 per cent of the ^{14}C-leucine which enters the two cell stage embryos is incorporated into PCA precipitable material during a

133

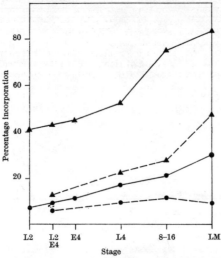

Fig. 2. Effects of cycloheximide (0·5 μg/ml.) on the rates of RNA and protein synthesis in cleavage stage mouse embryos. Embryos were incubated for 3 h at each stage in either 6 μCi/ml. ³H-5-uridine (●) or 0·6 μCi/ml. ¹⁴C-leucine (▲) in the presence (- - -) or absence (————) of cycloheximide.

3 h treatment. This level of incorporation increases only slightly through the four cell stage. Between the L4 and eight to sixteen cell stages there is a major increase in the rate of protein synthesis (23 per cent higher than the rate at the L4 stage). This increase coincides with a great increase in the numbers of cytoplasmic polyribosomes noted in ultrastructural studies[10,12], and is in agreement with autoradiographic data[2]. The rate of protein synthesis increases to 83 per cent incorporation at the morula stage. These rates of protein synthesis are not altered during the exposure to actinomycin D (either 0·0008 μg/ml. or 0·1 μg/ml., Fig. 1), except for a slight reduction at the two cell stage (0·1 μg/ml.) and stimulation at the two cell and four cell stages (0·0008 μg/ml.). Actinomycin treatment of 0·1 μg/ml., which almost completely blocks RNA synthesis at each stage, does not reduce the rate of protein synthesis (Fig. 1).

Cycloheximide (0·5 μg/ml.) treatment decreases the rate of protein synthesis by at least 30 per cent at all stages (Fig. 2), but does not interfere with development. (Regardless of the cleavage stage at which treatment is applied, reincubated embryos continue to form blastocysts which differentiate normally.) The reduction in the rate of protein synthesis (absolute decrease in percentage incorporation) is approximately the same at each stage, except for a slightly greater inhibition at the eight to sixteen cell stage (Fig. 2). In addition to this effect on protein synthesis, cycloheximide reduces the rate of RNA synthesis, leucine uptake and, to a lesser extent, uridine uptake (Figs. 2 and 3). In each of these cases, the reductions are greater at the morula stage than at the earlier stages.

More detailed information concerning the effects of

cycloheximide on RNA synthesis was obtained through sucrose density gradient analysis of drug-treated, ^{3}H-5-uridine labelled, morula stage embryos. Fig. 4 shows that the two major species of rRNA sediment at the same relative positions in both control and experimental gradient analyses. A quantitative analysis of the relative amount of 30–32S rRNA and 18S rRNA, in comparison with the total amount of new RNA synthesis (determined by

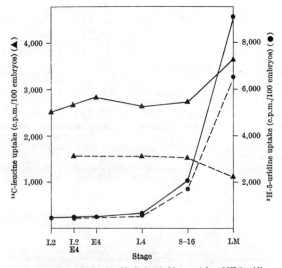

Fig. 3. Effects of cycloheximide (0·5 μg/ml.) on uptake of ^{3}H-5-uridine and ^{14}C-leucine by cleavage stage mouse embryos. The points on the graph represent the total uptake of precursors from the experiments shown in Fig. 2. The symbols are the same as those in Fig. 2.

perchloric acid (PCA) extraction), shows that although the cycloheximide treatment causes an 11 per cent reduction (15 per cent to 4·1 per cent) in rRNA synthesis, there is a reduction of RNA synthesis (PCA extraction) of 21 per cent. This latter reduction cannot be accounted for by the 11 per cent decrease in the rate of rRNA synthesis. Thus in cleavage stage mouse embryos, cycloheximide affects RNA synthesis in general, and is not specific for rRNA as opposed to reports on other systems[13].

135

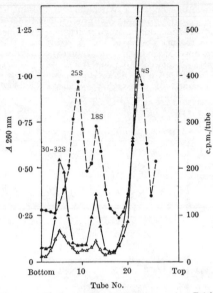

	Percentage 30–32S rRNA	Percentage 18S rRNA	Total PCA extracted RNA (percentage incorporation)
Control (▲)	10	5	30
Cycloheximide (△)	3	1	10

Fig. 4. Inhibition of morula stage RNA synthesis by cycloheximide (0·5 µg/ml., 3 h). Sucrose density gradient analysis. Techniques for labelling, collecting and storing the embryos are the same as those described in the text. 25S, 18S (wheat germ rRNA, Calbiochem) and 4S (stripped calf liver sRNA, General Biochemicals) were used for the absorbance reference peaks (●). Thawed embryos were lysed in 0·5 ml., 0·01 M Tris-HCl (pH 7·4), 1 per cent sodium dodecyl sulphate, 100 µg/ml. polyvinyl sulphate. The lysate was placed on top of a 16·5 ml., 5–20 per cent sucrose gradient (prepared in 0·01 M sodium acetate, pH 5·0, 0·1 M NaCl, 0·1 mM EDTA) and the tubes were centrifuged at 24,000 r.p.m. for 18 h, 20° C, in a Spinco L2-65 ultracentrifuge (SW 25·3 rotor). Nine drop fractions were collected from the bottom of the gradient, the absorbance at 260 nm recorded for each fraction, and radioactivity assayed in a Packard 'Tri-Carb' liquid scintillation counter. The amount of radioactivity under each rRNA peak is summated and expressed as a percentage of the total uptake of ³H-5-uridine by the embryos. The radioactivity at the top of the gradients is largely acid-soluble material. The data for total PCA extracted RNA, expressed as percentage incorporation, are derived from the experiments shown in Fig. 2.

In summary, the lower concentration of actinomycin D neither blocks cell division nor blastocyst differentiation when applied at the two cell or four cell stages. This is reasonable when one considers that rRNA synthesis is either non-detectable or at relatively low levels at these early stages[8,9,14], and may not be needed for early cleavage stage protein synthesis. The greater inhibition of RNA synthesis in the later stages probably reflects the normally increased rates of rRNA synthesis at these stages[8,9]. The inhibition of rRNA synthesis may be responsible for the blockage of blastocyst differentiation in embryos which were treated at the eight cell and morula stages.

The use of 0·1 µg/ml. of actinomycin D shows that concurrent RNA synthesis is not necessary for protein synthesis during mouse cleavage. This suggests that the messenger, transfer and ribosomal RNAs which are required for protein synthesis are stable for at least 3 h

136

at each stage. This same concentration of actinomycin D, however, blocks cell division. Although this blockage may be the result of the almost total inhibition of RNA synthesis, high concentrations of the drug are known to damage chromatin material[4,15]. This effect could also be responsible for the cessation of cell division.

The cycloheximide experiments show that normal rates of protein synthesis are necessary for the maintenance of the normal rates of RNA synthesis and leucine and uridine uptake. The time between the inhibition of protein synthesis and the inhibition of transport and RNA synthesis may reflect the size of the available pool of proteins required for these processes. In the present instance, the rates of RNA synthesis and the transport of amino-acids and nucleosides are reduced in less than 3 h. Thus in normal conditions the required proteins must be newly synthesized within a 3 h period. The greater inhibition of both RNA synthesis and transport of precursors at the later cleavage stages may be caused by an increasing demand for certain proteins which are involved in these activities[16-20]. It is likely that newly synthesized ribosomal proteins are among those proteins required at the later cleavage stages, for these stages are characterized by large increases in the production of rRNA[8,9], the appearance of many cytoplasmic polyribosomes[10] and the incorporation of ^{3}H-leucine into the nucleolus[2]. Further studies should clarify some of the interrelationships between RNA and protein synthesis in cleaving mouse embryos.

This work was supported by a research grant and a training grant from the US National Institutes of Health.

1 Thomson, J. L., and Biggers, J. D., *Exp. Cell Res.*, 41, 411 (1966).
2 Mintz, B., *J. Exp. Zool.*, 157, 85 (1964).
3 Skalko, R. G., and Morse, J. M. D., *Teratology*, 2, 47 (1969).
4 Silagi, S., *Exp. Cell Res.*, 32, 149 (1963).
5 Edwards, R. G., and Gates, A. H., *J. Endocrinol.*, 18, 292 (1959).
6 Brinster, R. L., *Exp. Cell Res.*, 32, 205 (1963).
7 Schmidt, G., and Thannhauser, S., *J. Biol. Chem.*, 161, 83 (1945).
8 Woodland, H. R., and Graham, C. F., *Nature*, 221, 327 (1969).
9 Ellem, K. A. O., and Gwatkin, R. B. L., *Develop. Biol.*, 18, 311 (1968).
10 Hillman, N. W., and Tasca, R. J., *Amer. J. Anat.* (in the press).
11 Perry, R. P., *Exp. Cell Res.*, 29, 400 (1963).
12 Hillman, N. W., and Tasca, R. J., *Proc. Twelfth Intern. Cong. Genetics, Tokyo*, Abstr. 7.5.1 (1968).
13 Jackson, L. G., and Studzinski, G. P., *Exp. Cell Res.*, 52, 408 (1968).
14 Monesi, V., and Salfi, V., *Exp. Cell Res.*, 46, 632 (1967).
15 Fautrez-Firlefyn, N., and Fautrez, J., *Intern. Rev. Cytol.*, 22, 171 (1967).
16 Busch, H., *Histones and Other Nuclear Proteins* (Academic Press, New York, 1965).
17 Chalkley, G. R., and Maurer, H. R., *Proc. US Nat. Acad. Sci.*, 54, 498 (1965).
18 Paul, J., and Gilmour, R. S., *J. Mol. Biol.*, 34, 305 (1968).
19 Mitchison, J. M., and Cummins, J. E., *J. Cell Sci.*, 1, 35 (1966).
20 Pardee, A. B., *Nat. Cancer Inst. Monograph.*, 27, 249 (1967).

THE UPTAKE OF HEXOSES BY PRE-IMPLANTATION MOUSE EMBRYOS *IN VITRO*

R. G. WALES AND R. L. BRINSTER

INTRODUCTION

During development of in-vitro techniques for the cultivation of mouse embryos at the pre-implantation stages of development, it was found that the late 2-cell embryo would not develop to the blastocyst when glucose was the sole energy source (Brinster, 1965a). On the other hand, 8-cell embryos would continue development when this substrate was provided (Brinster & Thomson, 1966). Recent studies using L-malate (Wales & Biggers, 1968) have indicated that the cell membrane undergoes a change in permeability to this substrate between the first and third cleavage divisions. This raises the question as to whether a similar change in permeability to glucose occurs at this time and is responsible for the difference in the ability of glucose to support development at these two stages.

In an attempt to throw light on this problem, the intracellular accumulation of glucose carbon has been studied at various stages in development. Some studies on the accumulation of galactose are also included.

MATERIALS AND METHODS

Mouse embryos were obtained from random-bred Swiss mice which had been superovulated by an intraperitoneal injection of 10 i.u. of serum gonadotrophin (Gestyl, Organon), followed 48 hr later by an intraperitoneal injection of 10 i.u. of chorionic gonadotrophin (Pregnyl, Organon) (Brinster, 1963). Successive developmental stages of the embryos were removed from the Fallopian tubes of mice at specific times after ovulation. The cumulus cells which surrounded unfertilized ova and single-cell embryos were removed by incubation in hyaluronidase solution (Brinster, 1965b). The basic medium used in the study and the method of washing the embryos free of substrate before incubation have been described previously (Wales & Biggers, 1968). For the studies of the uptake of substrates, incubations were carried out in tissue culture dishes containing a small drop of radio-active medium in 10 ml of light paraffin oil. In the first experiments, 200 to 300 2-cell embryos and eighty to 150 8-cell embryos were used for each treatment, but in later experiments fifty embryos/treatment were used for these stages and 150/treatment for 1-cell embryos. Incubations to study the production of carbon dioxide were set up in small test tubes as previously described (Brinster, 1967). For these experiments 300 to 400 2-cell embryos and 100 to 150 8-cell embryos were used.

The U-^{14}C-glucose (Nuclear Chicago Corp.) was diluted with basic diluent to give a concentration of 5·6 μmole/ml and a specific activity of 2·9 μc/μmole. For the experiment where a low concentration of glucose was used, the above solution was further diluted with basic, substrate-free medium to the desired concentration. The 1-^{14}C-galactose (Nuclear Chicago Corp.) was used at a concentration of 4·5 μmole/ml and a specific activity of 3·4 μc/μmole.

To measure the intracellular accumulation of substrate carbon, embryos, at the completion of incubation in the radio-active medium, were collected free of incubation medium and prepared for radio-active assay by liquid scintillation techniques as previously described (Wales & Biggers, 1968). Incubations at 5° C were carried out in a refrigerated room. After collection, the embryos were cooled to 5° C over 30 min in a diluent containing lactate (25 mM) and pyruvate (0·25 mM). They were then washed free of substrate at 5° C before incubation in the radio-active medium.

Samples of medium were taken for radio-assay at the completion of all incubations in order to determine the actual concentration of substrate present during the incubation period. These concentrations are given in the tables. The accumulation of substrate carbon was then calculated from the counts in the embryos and the specific activity of the substrate in the incubation medium. Where necessary, the data of Lewis & Wright (1935) were used as an estimate of the volume of the vitellus, to calculate the concentration of isotope in the embryo.

The method used to measure the production of carbon dioxide has been described previously (Brinster, 1967). After a 4-hr incubation, samples were acidified with 0·2 N-H_2SO_4 and the evolved carbon dioxide absorbed with 1 ml of 1 M p-(diisobutyl-cresoxyethoxyethyl)dimethyl benzyl ammonium hydroxide (hyamine hydroxide, Packard Instrument Company). The radio-activity was then assayed by liquid scintillation techniques.

RESULTS

The overall results for the accumulation of substrate carbon by 2- and 8-cell mouse embryos incubated in the presence of glucose (4·8 mM) are given in Table 1. After a 30-min incubation, 273×10^{-14} g atoms of substrate carbon

TABLE 1

ACCUMULATION OF SUBSTRATE CARBON BY MOUSE
EMBRYOS DURING A 30-MIN INCUBATION IN A DILUENT
CONTAINING 4·8 mM GLUCOSE AS SOLE ENERGY SOURCE

Stage of development	No. of observations	Substrate carbon accumulated ($g \, atoms \times 10^{-14}/embryo$)
2-cell	9	273 ± 10
8-cell	12	301 ± 9

Mean values ± standard errors of the means are given.

accumulated in 2-cell embryos, while in 8-cell embryos, 301×10^{-14} g atoms were found. The difference between 2- and 8-cell embryos was just significant ($t_{19} = 2·1$, $P = 0·05$). By comparison the amount of substrate carbon found in 1-cell embryos under similar conditions (Table 2) was low although not as

TABLE 2

UPTAKE OF GLUCOSE (3·8 mM) BY UNFERTILIZED AND
FERTILIZED MOUSE OVA DURING A 30-MIN INCUBATION
IN THE PRESENCE OR ABSENCE OF LACTATE (5 mM) AND
PYRUVATE (0·05 mM)

Stage of development	Lactate + pyruvate	Glucose carbon accumulated ($g \, atoms \times 10^{-14}/embryo$)	
		Rep 1	Rep 2
Unfertilized	−	14	13
	+	13	15
Fertilized	−	46	51
	+	40	44

low as that found in unfertilized ova. The addition of low levels of lactate and pyruvate to the incubation medium as a readily available alternative energy source did not increase the accumulation of glucose carbon by either fertilized or unfertilized ova.

The effect of varying conditions on the intra-cellular levels of glucose carbon in 2- and 8-cell embryos is shown in Tables 3, 4 and 5. A change in the incubation temperature from 37° C to 5° C almost completely eliminated any uptake of substrate carbon at both stages of development (Table 3). In the second experiment (Table 4), a glucose concentration of 0·5 mM, instead of 5 mM, resulted in a fall in the intracellular level of glucose carbon to 40% of that found with the higher concentration. However, with 0·5 mM glucose, the concentration of substrate carbon in the cell was 2·5 times that in the medium.

TABLE 3

COMPARISON OF INCUBATION AT $37°$ C AND $5°$ C FOR
30 MIN ON THE ACCUMULATION OF SUBSTRATE CARBON
BY MOUSE EMBRYOS IN A DILUENT CONTAINING 4·9 mM
GLUCOSE

Stage of development	Temperature of incubation (°C)	Substrate carbon accumulated (g atoms × 10⁻¹⁴/embryo)	
		Rep 1	Rep 2
2-cell	37	165	178
	5	4	2
8-cell	37	297	311
	5	6	9

By contrast, substrate carbon concentration was lower in the cell than in the medium when 5 mM glucose was added to the incubation medium.

A third experiment was carried out to study the effects of varying the time of

TABLE 4

EFFECT OF A CHANGE IN GLUCOSE CONCENTRATION ON
THE ACCUMULATION OF SUBSTRATE CARBON BY MOUSE
EMBRYOS

Stage of development	Glucose concentration (mM)	Substrate carbon accumulated	
		(i) g atoms × 10⁻¹⁴/embryo	(ii) μg atoms/ml
2-cell	5·0	261	17
	0·5	111	7
8-cell	4·7	327	24
	0·5	126	9

Mean values for two replicates are given.

incubation (Table 5). For 2-cell embryos, aliquots of two collections of embryos were incubated 3, 9, 27 and 81 min. In the case of 8-cell embryos, insufficient numbers of embryos were collected for all times to be studied at once and a

TABLE 5

ACCUMULATION OF SUBSTRATE CARBON DURING VARY-
ING PERIODS OF INCUBATION IN 5·1 mM GLUCOSE

Incubation time (min)	Substrate carbon accumulated (g atoms × 10⁻¹⁴/embryo)					
	2-cell		8-cell			
			Exp. 1		Exp. 2	
	Rep 1	Rep 2	Rep 1	Rep 2	Rep 1	Rep 2
3	53	60	68	60	–	–
9	137	122	172	158	–	–
27	248	248	319	281	245	336
81	286	393	–	–	519	615

complementary experiment comparing 27 and 81 min was carried out separately (see Table 5). Substrate carbon accumulated rapidly in 2-cell embryos during the first 9 min of incubation. Thereafter, the rate of its accumulation decreased. Its concentration doubled during the next 18 min and the levels at 81 min were only 40% above those at 27 min. At all times, there was more substrate carbon accumulation in 8-cell embryos than in 2-cell embryos, and the difference became greater as the time of incubation was increased. This was due to the fact that the rate of accumulation of substrate carbon in 8-cell embryos did not fall off as rapidly with time and the levels doubled between 27 and 81 min.

TABLE 6

METABOLISM OF HEXOSE CARBON BY MOUSE EMBRYOS INCUBATED IN A DILUENT CONTAINING 3·6 mM 1-^{14}C-GALACTOSE

Stage of development	Carbon one of galactose accumulated in 30 min		CO_2 produced from carbon one during 4-hr incubation	
	No. of observations	g atoms × 10^{-14}/ embryo	No. of observations	moles × 10^{-14}/ embryo
2-cell	4	41·1 ± 1·9	3	21·3 ± 18·0
8-cell	4	45·5 ± 1·4	3	89·7 ± 2·2

Mean values ± standard errors of the means are given.

In the final experiments, the uptake and utilization of 1-^{14}C-galactose by mouse embryos was investigated. The accumulation of substrate carbon and the production of carbon dioxide from carbon position one of galactose are shown in Table 6. The accumulation of carbon from position one of galactose

TABLE 7

UPTAKE OF 1-^{14}C-GALACTOSE (3·7 mM) BY MOUSE EMBRYOS DURING 30-MIN INCUBATION IN THE PRESENCE OR ABSENCE OF LACTATE (5 mM) PLUS PYRUVATE (0·05 mM)

Stage of development	Lactate+ pyruvate	Carbon one of galactose accumulated (g atoms × 10^{-14}/embryo)	
		Rep 1	Rep 2
2-cell	−	41	43
	+	46	41
8-cell	−	48	48
	+	52	53

was one-sixth the total accumulation of carbon from U-^{14}C-glucose. The levels in 8-cell embryos showed a tendency to be higher but the difference was not significant. On the other hand, the production of carbon dioxide by 8-cell embryos was higher than that from the 2-cell stage. In a further experiment (Table 7), the addition of low levels of lactate (5 mM) and pyruvate (0·05 mM) to the incubation medium did not significantly affect the accumulation of carbon one of galactose in either 2- or 8-cell embryos.

142

The effect of a combination of glucose and galactose on their respective accumulation was also studied. For each sample of embryos collected, equal numbers of embryos were transferred to four droplets of medium containing, respectively, radio-active glucose alone, radio-active glucose plus non-radio-active galactose, radio-active galactose alone and radio-active galactose plus non-radio-active glucose. By assay of the radio-activity incorporated into the

TABLE 8

ACCUMULATION OF HEXOSE CARBON BY MOUSE EMBRYOS INCUBATED 30 MIN IN A DILUENT CONTAINING GLUCOSE (4·8 mM) OR GALACTOSE (4·0 mM) ALONE AND IN COMBINATION

Stage of development	Total glucose carbon accumulated		Carbon one of galactose accumulated	
	− galactose	+ galactose	− glucose	+ glucose
2-cell	250	230	39	19**
8-cell	285	208**	44	22**

Values are expressed as g atoms × 10^{-14}/embryo and are the means of two replicates.
** Significant effect of combination on carbon accumulation, $P < 0.01$.

embryos in each droplet, the accumulation of substrate carbon from both glucose and galactose, alone or in combination, could be calculated. The results for two replicates at each stage of development (Table 8) showed that the addition of galactose decreased the accumulation of glucose carbon slightly. On the other hand, the intracellular level of galactose carbon was halved by the addition of glucose to the incubation medium.

DISCUSSION

In these studies a great change in the accumulation of substrate carbon from glucose occurred about the time of fertilization and first cleavage, but after this time there was only a slight change in substrate accumulation. In other studies, it has been found that carbon dioxide production from glucose continues to increase through all stages of development (Brinster, 1967). Wales & Whittingham (1968) have found no difference between 1- and 2-cell embryos in their oxidative utilization of lactate or pyruvate; thus the available evidence points either to rate of transport or to rate of glycolysis as the mechanism governing the production of energy from glucose in the embryos.

In the case of malic acid, a difference in permeability between 2- and 8-cell mouse embryos (Wales & Biggers, 1968) explains why this compound will support development only from the 8-cell stage. The position appears to be quite different for glucose, where similar amounts of glucose carbon accumulate in the cell at the 2- and 8-cell stage during a 30-min incubation. At the same time, the increase in the accumulation of substrate carbon with time was far greater for 8- than 2-cell mouse embryos, indicating that differences exist between 2- and 8-cell mouse embryos in their metabolism of glucose. However, it is not clear if it is the greater accumulation of metabolic products in 8-cell embryos or the greater oxidative utilization of glucose by 8- as compared to 2-cell embryos (Brinster, 1967) that is responsible for the ability of glucose to maintain development only after the third cell division.

Incubation of the embryos in glucose at the specific activity used resulted in the accumulation of approximately 3 d.p.m./embryo. At such a low level of radio-activity, it was impossible to make even a preliminary fractionation of the substrate carbon accumulated within the cell. Thus the nature of the accumulated products is a matter for debate. No doubt some of the carbon accumulates as the parent substrate. At the same time, some will have entered the carbon pools of the embryo and the net accumulation of isotope will depend on the size and number of these pools and on the rates of reaction repleting and depleting them. Brinster (1967) has indicated that the pentose shunt is operative in mouse embryos at this stage of development, and thus some of the carbon accumulated may arise from synthetic reactions involving this pathway. In addition, Wales & Whittingham (1968) have found that there is intracellular accumulation of metabolic products following decarboxylation of pyruvate or lactate in the mouse embryo.

The mechanism of transfer of monosaccharides across membranes differs from tissue to tissue. Glucose uptake has been described as active transport in the isolated intestine of the guinea-pig (Riklis, Haber & Quastel, 1958) and in suspensions of isolated rat intestinal epithelial cells (Stern & Jensen 1966), but in erythrocytes and muscle has been explained on the basis of an exchange diffusion (Mawe & Hempling, 1965; Park, Reinwein, Henderson, Cadenas & Morgan, 1959) involving a membrane carrier but lacking an energy-consuming link. In embryos, elucidation of the mechanism of transport is made difficult because few cells are able to be harvested for study and as mentioned above it was impossible to identify what portion of the intracellular carbon accumulating is the parent substrate. However, a very substantial increase in the specific activity of the substrate may make it possible to recover sufficient isotope to allow identification of the materials accumulated in the embryo and thus to determine if an active transport system exists in embryos for the movement of glucose across the cell membrane. At the same time, the virtual absence of substrate in embryos incubated at 5° C indicates that little, if any, of the substrate enters the cell by diffusion.

Galactose, the naturally occurring isomer of glucose, behaves as a non-utilizable substance in most animal tissues (see Levine & Goldstein, 1955) and has been used as an indicator of hexose transport in spermatozoa (Flipse, 1962). The competition between glucose and galactose in embryos is similar to that reported in guinea-pig intestine (Riklis, Haber & Quastel, 1958), tissue culture cells (Rickenberg & Maio, 1960) and rabbit kidney cortex (Krane & Crane, 1959). However, the finding that mouse embryos utilize galactose to some extent makes it impossible at the present stage of our knowledge to differentiate between competition for uptake as is found in other tissues and competition for entry of metabolic products into the common carbon pools.

ACKNOWLEDGMENTS

This work was supported by grants from the Population Council and the

National Science Foundation (GB 4465). One of the authors (R.G.W.) is indebted to the Population Council and the Australian Wool Board for financial assistance while on sabbatical leave from the University of Sydney.

REFERENCES

BRINSTER, R. L. (1963) A method for *in vitro* cultivation of mouse ova from two-cell to blastocyst. *Expl Cell Res.* 32, 205.

BRINSTER, R. L. (1965a) Studies on the development of mouse embryos *in vitro*. II. The effect of energy source. *J. exp. Zool.* 158, 59.

BRINSTER, R. L. (1965b) Lactic dehydrogenase activity in the preimplanted mouse embryo. *Biochim. biophys. Acta*, 110, 439.

BRINSTER, R. L. (1967) Carbon dioxide production from glucose by the preimplantation mouse embryo. *Expl Cell Res.* 47, 271.

BRINSTER, R. L. & THOMSON, J. L. (1966) Development of eight-cell mouse embryos *in vitro*. *Expl Cell Res.* 42, 308.

FLIPSE, R. J. (1962) Metabolism of bovine semen. XII. Galactose as an indicator of hexose transport by bovine spermatozoa. *J. Dairy Sci.* 45, 1083.

KRANE, S. M. & CRANE, R. K. (1959) The accumulation of D-galactose against a concentration gradient by slices of rabbit kidney cortex. *J. biol. Chem.* 234, 211.

LEVINE, R. & GOLDSTEIN, M. S. (1955) On the mechanism of action of insulin. *Recent Prog. Horm. Res.* 11, 343.

LEWIS, W. H. & WRIGHT, E. S. (1935) On the early development of the mouse egg. *Contrib. Embryol.* 25, 113.

MAWE, R. C. & HEMPLING, H. G. (1965) The exchange of C^{14} glucose across the membrane of the human erythrocyte. *J. cell. comp. Physiol.* 66, 95.

PARK, C. R., REINWEIN, D., HENDERSON, M. J., CADENAS, E. & MORGAN, H. E. (1959) The action of insulin on the transport of glucose through cell membranes. *Am. J. Med.* 26, 674.

RICKENBERG, H. V. & MAIO, J. J. (1960) *The transport of galactose by mammalian tissue culture cells*. In: Membrane Transport and Metabolism, p. 409. Eds. A. Kleinzeller and A. Kotyk. Academic Press, London.

RIKLIS, E., HABER, B. & QUASTEL, J. H. (1958) Absorption of mixtures of sugars by isolated surviving guinea pig intestine. *Can. J. Biochem. Physiol.* 36, 373.

STERN, B. K. & JENSEN, W. E. (1966) Active transport of glucose by suspensions of isolated rat intestinal epithelial cells. *Nature, Lond.* 209, 5025.

WALES, R. G. & BIGGERS, J. D. (1968) The permeability of two- and eight-cell mouse embryos to L-malic acid. *J. Reprod. Fert.* 15, 103.

WALES, R. G. & WHITTINGHAM, D. G. (1967) A comparison of the uptake and utilization of lactate and pyruvate by one- and two-cell mouse embryos. *Biochim. biophys. Acta*, 148, 703.

THE FIXATION OF CARBON DIOXIDE BY THE
EIGHT-CELL MOUSE EMBRYO

R. G. WALES, P. QUINN AND R. N. MURDOCH

Mouse embryos require the presence of a bicarbonate buffer system for their development *in vitro*. The energy requirements for oocyte maturation and early zygote development prompted Biggers, Whittingham & Donahue (1967) to suggest that the fixation of carbon dioxide may play a rôle in the energy metabolism of the early embryo. The present study was undertaken in an attempt to demonstrate this reaction in the eight-cell mouse embryo.

For each experiment, 400 eight-cell mouse embryos were flushed from the reproductive tracts of superovulated female albino mice. The basic medium was Krebs-Ringer bicarbonate containing 25 mM-sodium DL lactate, 0·25 mM-sodium pyruvate, 0·01 mM-sodium ketoglutarate, 0·01 mM-sodium malate, 0·01 mM-sodium citrate, 1 mg/ml bovine serum albumin, 60 μg/ml penicillin, 50 μg/ml streptomycin. After washing by transfer through two changes (2 ml each) of this medium, the embryos were cultured in 20 μl droplets of medium (forty embryos/drop) containing $NaH^{14}CO_3$ (specific activity 10 mCi/m-mole) in a 35-mm diameter plastic culture dish (Falcon Plastics) containing 3 ml light paraffin oil. The culture dish was cemented in a glass petri dish of approximately 27-ml volume. Sufficient radio-active bicarbonate, of the same specific activity as that in the culture medium, was pipetted into one side of the glass petri dish to produce a 5% CO_2 atmosphere in the dish after acidification and 0·2 ml of 6 N-H_2SO_4 was pipetted into the opposite side of the dish. The lid of the petri dish was sealed and the dish tipped slightly to mix the acid with the bicarbonate to release carbon dioxide.

After a 24-hr period of culture at 37° C, all the developed embryos were separated from the medium as previously described (Wales & Biggers, 1968). The medium was also collected and both embryos and medium were acidified with 0·1 ml 2 N-H_2SO_4 and placed in a closed container containing 2 N-NaOH for 24 hr to absorb liberated carbon dioxide. After neutralization with NaOH, a small aliquot was taken for radio-assay and the remainder was fractionated to determine the amount of label in the acid-soluble, protein and lipid fractions as described below.

A 50-μl sample of sheep serum was added to both embryos and medium to act as carrier for the labelled compounds. Protein was precipitated with 2·5% perchloric acid. After washing the precipitate four times with 20% trichloroacetic acid, it was extracted with chloroform–ether (1:1). The acid-soluble fraction was fractionated into basic, neutral and acidic compounds by passing it through a column of cation exchange resin followed by an anion exchange resin. Full details of the method will be published elsewhere.

In a preliminary experiment, 400 eight-cell embryos which had been inactivated by incubation for 30 min in phosphate-buffered saline containing 10% formalin, were kept for 24 hr in radio-active bicarbonate in the same manner as the living embryos. After collection and acidification, a total of 7 counts/min was found in these dead embryos. This compares with 16,000 counts/min when the same number of live embryos was cultured. In addition, the medium in which the formalin-killed embryos were kept contained the same number of counts after acidification and extraction as a control sample of unincubated medium similarly treated. Both contained 0·005% of the added isotope and correction was made for these background counts in calculating the net incorporation of isotope in the following experiments.

Table 1 shows the results of the experiments to measure the incorporation of carbon from bicarbonate by eight-cell embryos during 24 hr in culture. In the three experiments, an average of 94% of embryos developed into morulae or

TABLE 1

INCORPORATION OF CARBON FROM SODIUM BICARBONATE BY EIGHT-CELL
MOUSE EMBRYOS DURING 24 HR IN CULTURE

Fraction assayed	Replicate no.	Carbon incorporated (μg atoms $\times 10^{-8}$/embryo)					
		Total	Acid soluble compounds			Protein fraction	Lipid fraction
			Acidic	Basic	Neutral		
Embryos	1	323	197	113	13	93	5
	2	313	172	128	13	70	6
	3	426	251	162	17	111	11
	Mean	354	207	134	14	91	7
Medium	1	175	114	35	26	0	0
	2	252	164	63	25	0	0
	3	249	154	67	30	0	0
	Mean	225	144	55	27	0	0

early blastocysts. Most of the isotope incorporated into the embryos was present in the acid-soluble fraction. Of this, 60% was incorporated into acidic compounds, 38% into basic compounds and there was a minor labelling of the neutral fraction. In addition, there was substantial incorporation into the protein of the embryo and a minor labelling of lipids.

Incorporation into the acid-soluble fraction of the medium was also substantial and as the major portion of the label was present in acidic compounds, an aliquot was applied to a column of silicic acid and the carboxylic acids eluted with hexane–butanol mixtures (O'Shea & Wales, 1968). Approximately 50% of the labelled acidic compounds were eluted in the peak corresponding to lactate, and other smaller peaks corresponding to acetate, malate, keto-glutarate and citrate were also seen. Probably, this accumulation of radio-active products in the medium only reflects the leakage of certain metabolic intermediates from the embryo during culture and their trapping in the substrate pool of the medium. When aliquots of the acid-soluble fraction of embryos were chromatographed in a similar fashion, only a small proportion of the isotope applied was eluted and no radio-active peak corresponding to lactate was found.

The results demonstrate a substantial gain in carbon by the embryo through fixation of carbon dioxide from the surroundings. A similar amount of carbon-one of pyruvate is accumulated in the embryo during this period when 0·5 mM-pyruvate is present as sole substrate (R. G. Wales & D. G. Whittingham, unpublished observations). This suggests that the main route of entry for carbon-one of pyruvate into the carbon pool of the embryo is by the conversion of pyruvate to oxaloacetate. Thus, in addition to maintaining a suitable hydrogen ion concentration in the incubation medium, bicarbonate buffer supplies the carbon for this conversion. However, bicarbonate may play some further function in the developing embryo as no development of eight-cell embryos to blastocysts occurred when oxaloacetate was substituted for pyruvate in the medium and the zwitterionic buffer N-2-hydroxyethylpiperazine-N'-2-ethanesulphonic acid was used.

The authors are grateful to Professor C. W. Emmens for his interest and criticism. The work was aided by a grant from the Australian Research Grants Committee. One of us (P.Q.) was supported by an Australian Wool Board Post-graduate studentship.

REFERENCES

BIGGERS, J. D., WHITTINGHAM, D. G. & DONAHUE, R. P. (1967) The pattern of energy metabolism in the mouse oocyte and zygote. *Proc. natn. Acad. Sci. U.S.A.* **58,** 560.

O'SHEA, T. & WALES, R. G. (1968) Metabolism of [1-14C]sodium lactate and [2-14C]sodium lactate by ram spermatozoa. *J. Reprod. Fert.* **15,** 337.

WALES, R. G. & BIGGERS, J. D. (1968) The permeability of two- and eight-cell mouse embryos to L-malic acid. *J. Reprod. Fert.* **15,** 103.

THE PERMEABILITY OF TWO- AND EIGHT-CELL MOUSE EMBRYOS TO L-MALIC ACID

R. G. WALES AND J. D. BIGGERS

INTRODUCTION

Biggers, Gwatkin & Brinster (1962) showed that complete development of the mouse zygote to a blastocyst *in vitro* only occurred in organ cultures of Fallopian tubes. At the time these organ culture studies were done, only late 2-cell mouse embryos would develop into blastocysts completely *in vitro*, provided lactate was incorporated in the medium (Whitten, 1957). These results provided indirect evidence that cleavage in the mouse is dependent on the maternal environment. More recent studies have shown that development of the late 2-cell mouse embryo to the blastocyst (Brinster, 1963), and the zygote to the early 2-cell stage (Whittingham & Biggers, 1967), can occur in a simple chemically-defined medium, only if an energy source is present. Only in the intermitotic period between the first and second cleavages is some unknown Fallopian tube factor involved. Thus, there is strong circumstantial evidence that Fallopian tube secretions supply at least an exogenous energy source to the embryo throughout cleavage.

The fact that cleaving mouse embryos require an exogenous energy source raises questions as to what energy sources can be used and how they are assimilated. Studies on the nutritional requirements of the cleaving mouse embryo *in vitro* indicate that the energetics of early development are complex. The spectrum of compounds which can be utilized by the late 2-cell embryo is narrow, restricted to the four compounds: lactate, pyruvate, phosphoenolpyruvate and oxaloacetate (Brinster, 1963). By the 8-cell stage, however, several other compounds, such as glucose, malate, α-ketoglutarate and citrate can be used (Whitten, 1957; Brinster & Thomson, 1966). Two alternative mechanisms may be invoked to explain these findings. Either the energy source cannot enter the embryo until a certain stage of development is reached because of permeability barriers, or the energy source enters the early embryo, but the necessary metabolic pathways for its utilization do not develop until later. Studies of the uptake of $U^{14}C$-L-malate by 2- and 8-cell mouse embryos have shown that the cell membrane becomes permeable to the compound between the first and third cleavage divisions. The results are reported in this paper.

MATERIALS AND METHODS

Mouse embryos were obtained from random-bred Swiss mice superovulated by the intraperitoneal injection of 10 i.u. of serum gonadotrophin (Gestyl, Organon), followed 48 hr later by the intraperitoneal injection of 10 i.u. of chorionic gonadotrophin (Pregnyl, Organon) (Brinster, 1963). Two-cell embryos were flushed from the Fallopian tubes of mated females 44 to 48 hr after the second injection, while 8-cell embryos were recovered from the Fallopian tubes and upper third of the uterus approximately 24 hr later.

The basic medium used in the study was Krebs–Ringer bicarbonate containing 1 mg/ml of crystalline bovine serum albumen, 100 i.u./ml of penicillin and 50 μg/ml of streptomycin. Where substrates were added to the medium, isotonicity was maintained by decreasing the sodium chloride content of the medium. For recovery and preliminary handling of the embryos, 25 mM sodium lactate and 0·25 mM sodium pyruvate were added as an energy source (Brinster, 1965). Following collection, the embryos were washed twice by transferring in a minimum volume through two changes of substrate-free medium (3 ml). Following the second wash, the embryos were collected in a minimum of substrate-free medium, transferred to a medium containing U-^{14}C-L-malate (1·7 mM and specific activity 4·4 μc/mole) and incubated at 37° C for 30 min with air:carbon dioxide (95:5) as the gas phase. Between 150 and 250 2-cell embryos, and between ninety and 110 8-cell embryos, were incubated for each treatment. In the first tests embryological watch glasses containing 0·5 ml of the malate medium covered with 2 ml of light paraffin oil were used. However, in all subsequent experiments, incubations were carried out in tissue culture dishes containing 0·1 ml of malate medium as a droplet in 10 ml of light paraffin oil (Brinster, 1963). This latter method was more convenient and conserved isotope. A preliminary trial showed that embryos could be incubated 30 min in the malate medium without loss of viability, as gauged by subsequent development into blastocysts.

A method used by Wales & O'Shea (1966) for the measurement of intracellular constituents of spermatozoa was adopted for the rapid recovery of the embryos from the radio-active malate medium. A 2·6-ml Pichler-Spikes type centrifuge tube with a uniform bore of 2 mm in the capillary tip was used

(Owens-Illinois Glass Co.). The bottom 0·5 cm (approximately 16 μl) was filled with 10% w/v sucrose solution containing 1% (v/v) formalin, and the remaining narrow portion of the tube (2 cm) was filled with isotonic sucrose. Above this, approximately 1 ml of non-radio-active malate medium (1·7 mM malate) was pipetted into the wide portion of the tube. At the completion of incubation in the radio-active malate, the embryos were transferred in a minimum volume of medium to the top of the non-radio-active medium and immediately centrifuged at 500 *g* for 3 min. The non-radio-active medium thus acted as an initial dilutor of the highly active incubation medium before centrifuging the embryos through the sucrose rinse.

After centrifugation, the supernatant medium was removed, the inner surface of the wide portion of the centrifuge tube wiped with absorbent tissue, rinsed with 1 ml of non-radio-active diluent and again wiped dry. The sucrose column was then carefully removed to within 1 cm of the base of the tube. The next 0·5 cm of sucrose was transferred to a scintillation vial to act as a background count for the embryos. The bottom of the tube (0·5 cm) was then removed and

TABLE 1

RADIO-ACTIVITY IN SUCCEEDING 16 μl ALIQUOTS OF THE SUCROSE RINSE AND IN EQUIVALENT AMOUNTS OF THE SUPERNATANT AND INCUBATION MEDIUM AFTER CENTRIFUGING MOUSE EMBRYOS

Stage of development	Radio-activity							
	Medium	Supernatant	Sucrose aliquots					
			1	2	3	4	5	6
2-cell embryo	114,757	7,629	21	4	2	1	0	11
8-cell embryo	124,733	4,379	15	2	2	2	0	64

Radio-activity is expressed as counts/min/aliquot corrected for background (26·8 counts/min). Following centrifugation and removal of the supernatant, succeeding aliquots of the sucrose rinse were withdrawn from the capillary tip of the centrifuge tube and assayed for radio-activity. The sucrose aliquots are numbered 1 to 6 from supernatant interface to base and aliquot number 6 contains the embryos.

transferred with its contents to a scintillation vial. Radio-activity was assayed by liquid scintillation techniques using toluene containing 0·5% 2,5-diphenyl-oxazole (PPO) and 0·03% 1-4-bis-2(4-methyl-5-phenyloxazolyl)-benzene (dimethyl POPOP) as scintillator. All samples were first dried, then incubated in 1 ml of 1 M methyl dodecyl benzyl trimethyl ammonium hydroxide (Hyamine hydroxide) before the addition of 10 ml of scintillator. Samples of low activity were counted for sufficient time to ensure accuracy. For each treatment a sample of incubation medium was assayed for radio-activity and the results used to determine the concentration of malate after the introduction of the embryos. The amount of intracellular substrate, expressed as μatoms of substrate carbon/embryo was calculated from the counts in the embryos, corrected for background and the specific activity of the incubation medium.

The distribution of isotope in the sucrose rinse, as shown in Table 1, indicates that the method effectively washes embryos free of radio-active medium. Little isotope was detected in the sucrose and the counts in the lower portion were

151

equal to those obtained with a standard background. Thus the mean count for the sucrose overlying the embryo fraction in all experiments was 26·8 (SE = 0·34, 32 observations) compared with a mean count of 26·8 (SE = 0·15, 8 observations) for a standard background.

To measure ^{14}C-carbon dioxide production, embryos were incubated in 0·1 ml of radio-active malate medium covered with a thin layer of light paraffin oil. Following incubation for 3 hr in sealed vials that had been flushed with air: carbon dioxide (95:5), metabolism was terminated by the injection of 0·1 ml of 0·2 N H_2SO_4 and the evolved carbon dioxide absorbed with 0·2 ml of 2 N NaOH. The absorbed carbon dioxide was precipitated as barium carbonate, collected on a filter disc, washed and quantitatively transferred to a scintillation vial in 2 ml of ethanol. The precipitate was dispersed in 10 ml of scintillator with the aid of an ultrasonic disintegrator and suspended with a thixotropic gel powder (Carb-O-Sil, Packard Instrument Company). As a consistent amount of radio-active carbon dioxide was collected from samples of the malate medium treated in this way, blanks containing no embryos were used as controls.

RESULTS

The level of intracellular substrate carbon in normal 2- and 8-cell mouse embryos incubated in $U^{14}C$-malate is shown in Table 2. There was little accumu-

TABLE 2

THE ACCUMULATION OF SUBSTRATE CARBON BY
MOUSE EMBRYOS DURING A 30-MIN INCUBATION
IN A DILUENT CONTAINING L-MALATE

Stage of development	No. of observations	Substrate carbon accumulated ($\mu gatoms \times 10^{-8}/embryo$)
2-cell	4	7·3 ± 2·9
8-cell	7	56·2 ± 5·0

Mean values ± standard errors of the means are given.

lation of substrate in 2-cell embryos following a 30-min incubation and the values represent counts only 57% higher than the corresponding background. On the other hand, significant amounts of substrate accumulated in 8-cell embryos and values were approximately eight times those found at the earlier stage in development.

The production of carbon dioxide from malate by 2- and 8-cell embryos was also measured. Two samples of 8-cell embryos produced 350×10^{-8} μmole and 420×10^{-8} μmole of carbon dioxide per embryo, respectively, during a 3-hr incubation. However, no carbon dioxide was produced by either of two samples of 2-cell embryos under similar conditions.

To examine the effect of removal of the zona pellucida on the accumulation of substrate carbon, 2- and 8-cell mouse embryos were collected. Before washing and incubation, half of each sample was incubated in a 0·25% solution of Pronase in phosphate buffered saline, containing 1% polyvinylpyrrolidone (pH 7·6) until the zona pelludica was digested (Mintz, 1962; Gwatkin, 1963).

The uptake of malate by these cells was then compared with that of the remaining untreated embryos (Table 3). Although the results are somewhat variable it seems that Pronase treatment had no effect on 2-cell embryos. In contrast, the accumulation of substrate by 8-cell embryos was significantly depressed by this treatment ($t_{(2)} = 7.7$, $0.01 < P < 0.05$).

TABLE 3

EFFECT OF REMOVING THE ZONA PELLUCIDA WITH
PRONASE ON THE AMOUNT OF SUBSTRATE CARBON
IN MOUSE EMBRYOS INCUBATED IN L-MALATE

Stage of development	Replicates	Substrate carbon accumulated (μgatoms $\times 10^{-8}$/embryo)	
		Untreated control	Pronase treated
2-cell	1	3.5	4.1
	2	15.4	3.6
	3	5.2	4.8
8-cell	1	69.5	40.4
	2	53.3	21.8
	3	77.6	34.8

The effect of varying the concentration of malate on the accumulation of substrate carbon by 8-cell embryos is shown in Table 4. A decrease in the concentration of malate during incubation from 1.17μmole/ml to 0.117μmole/ml caused a small (25%) decrease in the accumulation of substrate carbon by the embryos.

The uptake of malate by 8-cell embryos at low temperature was examined in the next experiment. After collection, the embryos were divided into three equal groups in separate embryological watch glasses containing 1 ml of medium

TABLE 4

THE EFFECT OF A CHANGE IN MALATE CON-
CENTRATION ON THE ACCUMULATION OF
SUBSTRATE CARBON BY 8-CELL MOUSE
EMBRYOS

Malate concentration (μmole/ml)	Substrate carbon accumulated (μgatoms $\times 10^{-8}$/embryo)	
	Rep 1	Rep 2
1.17	35.9	40.8
0.117	24.0	32.0

covered with 2 ml of light paraffin oil. Two groups were slowly cooled to 5° C over 30 min by standing in a shallow dish of water in a refrigerated room while the third was maintained at 37° C. A preliminary trial indicated that embryos so cooled showed no loss of viability as gauged by their subsequent development into blastocysts. One of the cooled groups was re-warmed for washing and incubation with the control, uncooled group. The other cooled group was washed

153

twice, incubated 30 min in the presence of radio-active malate and separated from the incubation medium, all at 5° C. The results for two replicates (Table 5) showed that the accumulation of substrate carbon was greatly depressed by incubation in malate at 5° C and was similar to that found in 2-cell embryos. On the other hand, embryos incubated in malate at 37° C, after cooling, accumulated substrate carbon as readily as the controls.

TABLE 5

EFFECT OF INCUBATION IN L-MALATE AT 5° C ON THE
AMOUNT OF SUBSTRATE CARBON IN 8-CELL MOUSE
EMBRYOS

Pretreatment	Temperature of incubation	Substrate carbon accumulated ($\mu gatoms \times 10^{-8}/embryo$)	
		Rep 1	Rep 2
Nil (control)	37° C	58·1	47·7
Cooled to 5° C	37° C	54·9	44·4
Cooled to 5° C	5° C	14·5	8·9

An attempt was made to block the uptake of malate by 8-cell mouse embryos with ouabain, an inhibitor of sodium–potassium dependent adenosine triphosphatase important in active transport of some substances across cell membranes (see Repke (1964) for a review).

The accumulation of substrate carbon by 8-cell mouse embryos in the presence of varying concentrations of ouabain was compared with that of control incubations containing no ouabain. The results (Table 6) indicate that

TABLE 6

EFFECT OF OUABAIN ON THE AMOUNT OF
SUBSTRATE CARBON IN 8-CELL MOUSE
EMBRYOS INCUBATED IN L-MALATE

Ouabain concentration (M)	Substrate carbon accumulated ($\mu gatoms \times 10^{-8}/embryo$)		
	Rep 1	Rep 2	Rep 3
0	44	44	52
10^{-7}	28	37	50
10^{-6}	56	37	—
10^{-5}	36	36	—

there is no effect of ouabain on the amount of intracellular substrate carbon during the 30-min incubation period.

DISCUSSION

UTILIZATION OF L-MALATE

Brinster (1966) has shown that NAD-dependent malic dehydrogenase is present in both 2- and 8-cell embryos and that oxaloacetate is able to support development at both stages (Brinster, 1965; Brinster & Thomson, 1966). Thus, it would be expected that, if malate could penetrate the cell wall of the 2-cell embryo, it would be utilized provided there was no inhibition of the dehydrogenase *in vivo*. However, it has been shown that malate will not support development at this stage (Brinster, 1965) and, in the present studies, oxidative utilization of malate by 2-cell embryos could not be demonstrated. In addition, the almost complete absence of substrate carbon in embryos at this stage indicates that there is no uptake of the substrate rather than an enzymic inhibition.

By comparison, there were consistently higher concentrations of isotopically labelled carbon in 8-cell embryos incubated in the presence of $U^{14}C$-malate, and a significant production of labelled carbon dioxide during incubation in its presence. These findings, plus the fact that a proportion of these embryos continue to develop with malate as sole substrate (Brinster & Thompson, 1966), indicate that this compound penetrates the 8-cell embryo and is utilized by oxidative pathways.

If 138,000 μ^3 is assumed to be the mean volume of the 8-cell mouse embryo (from data of Lewis & Wright, 1935), the values presented in Table 4 would give concentrations of intracellular substrate carbon of 2·78 and 2·02 μgatoms/ml when the extracellular values were 4·68 μgatoms/ml and 0·47 μgatoms/ml respectively. If the majority of substrate carbon in the cell was malate, the latter figure could indicate that uptake occurs against a concentration gradient. However, as very low levels of labelled substrate carbon were found even in 8-cell embryos, it was impossible to identify positively the intracellular constituent accumulating.

In the renal tubule it has been shown that three polycarboxylic acids of the tricarboxylic acid cycle, namely malate, α-ketoglutarate and citrate, are reabsorbed by active transport probably via a common mechanism (Vishwakarma & Miller, 1963). These three acids will not support the development of 2-cell mouse embryos but will support development of 8-cell stages (Brinster & Thomson, 1966). The present studies indicate that malate enters the 8-cell embryo by an active process. A change of substrate concentration in the incubation medium had a minor effect on the intracellular accumulation of substrate carbon whereas incubation at 5° C inhibited the accumulation. However, ouabain had no effect and it is unlikely therefore that the uptake of malate is linked to the sodium–potassium dependent adenosine triphosphatase as has been found for some non-electrolytes in other tissues (see Csaky, 1965).

The lack of accumulation of substrate carbon by 2-cell embryos during incubations in malate is not due to the impermeability of the zona pellucida at this stage. It has been shown that in the rabbit, rat and hamster the zona is permeable to substances with a molecular weight of at least 1200 (Austin & Lovelock, 1958) and, in the present experiments, removal of the zona by Pronase did not increase the uptake by 2-cell embryos. The effect of Pronase on the uptake of malate by 8-cell embryos is probably due to an effect of the non-specific proteolytic enzyme on cell constituents decreasing active uptake rather than to a direct effect of the removal of the zona pellucida freeing isotopic malate trapped in the perivitelline space. The tendency of some blastomeres to separate during treatment with this enzyme indicates that even with due precautions, there is some effect of the enzyme on the cell surface.

155

The work on the nutritional requirements of mouse embryos referred to in the introduction to this paper shows that the cleaving embryo is dependent on an exogenous supply of energy. Moreover, an increasing number of compounds can be used as development proceeds. The work described in the present paper has allowed us to identify more specifically one mechanism, namely a change in permeability, which may be involved in regulating development. Since active transport seems to be concerned in the uptake of malate by the mouse embryo the activation of a membrane-linked enzyme may be involved. The work of Fridhandler (1961) on the rabbit showed that initially the pentose phosphate pathway is the main route of energy metabolism, which is later replaced by the Emden-Myerhoff pathway. Thus, the joint evidence shows that more than one type of change in biochemical function may occur during cleavage in mammalian embryos. Cleavage, therefore, is not merely six to seven mitotic divisions in which a relatively undistinguished cytoplasm is shared out among the nuclei until some 64 to 128 cells are produced.

Although the ovum of a marine organism like *Arbacia* is very similar in size to the mouse ovum, there are at least two crucial differences in the mechanisms involved in cleavage of the two species. First, *Arbacia* readily cleave in artificial sea water which is devoid of an exogenous energy source (Shapiro, 1941), whereas a mouse requires an exogenous source of energy. Secondly, strong evidence exists that cleavage of the *Arbacia* egg until gastrulation is regulated by messenger RNA, which is performed in the oocyte (Gross & Cousineau, 1964), whereas, in the mouse, studies on the effect of actinomycin D on cleavage suggest that some synthesis of messenger RNA is necessary even at the 2-cell stage (Thomson & Biggers, 1966). Conclusive evidence of gene action during cleavage in the mouse is provided by two mutants (t^1 and t^{12}) which are lethal during cleavage in the homozygous state (Gluecksohn-Schoenheimer, 1938; Smith, 1956). In addition, the work of Fridhandler (1961) in the rabbit together with the demonstration that an active transport mechanism for the uptake of malate develops after the second cleavage may indicate that the differential reading of the genome begins early in cleavage.

ACKNOWLEDGMENTS

This work was aided by grants from the Population Council and the National Science Foundation (Grant No. GB 4465). One of the authors (R.G.W.) is also indebted to the Population Council for the provision of a fellowship while on sabbatical leave from the Department of Veterinary Physiology, University of Sydney, Australia.

REFERENCES

AUSTIN, C. R. & LOVELOCK, J. E. (1958) Permeability of rabbit, rat and hamster egg membranes. *Expl Cell Res.* 15, 260.
BIGGERS, J. D., GWATKIN, R. B. L. & BRINSTER, R. L. (1962) Development of mouse embryos in organ cultures of fallopian tubes on a chemically defined medium. *Nature, Lond.* 194, 747.
BRINSTER, R. L. (1963) A method for *in vitro* cultivation of mouse ova from two-cell to blastocyst. *Expl Cell Res.* 32, 205.

BRINSTER, R. L. (1965) Studies on the development of mouse embryos *in vitro*. IV. Interaction of energy sources. *J. Reprod. Fert.* **10**, 227.

BRINSTER, R. L. (1966) Malic dehydrogenase activity in the pre-implantation mouse embryo. *Expl Cell Res.* **43**, 131.

BRINSTER, R. L. & THOMSON, J. L. (1966) Development of eight-cell mouse embryos *in vitro*. *Expl Cell Res.* **42**, 308.

CSAKY, T. Z. (1965) Transport through biological membranes. *A. Rev. Physiol.* **27**, 415.

FRIDHANDLER, L. (1961) Pathways of glucose metabolism in fertilized rabbit ova at various pre-implantation stages. *Expl Cell Res.* **22**, 303.

GLUECKSOHN-SCHOENHEIMER, S. (1938) Time of death of lethal homozygotes in the T (Brachyury) series in the mouse. *Proc. Soc. exp. Biol. Med.* **39**, 267.

GROSS, P. R. & COUSINEAU, G. H. (1964) Macromolecule synthesis and the influence of actinomycin on early development. *Expl Cell Res.* **33**, 368.

GWATKIN, R. B. L. (1963) Effect of viruses on early mammalian development. I. Action of Mengo encephalitis virus on mouse ova cultivated *in vitro*. *Proc. natn. Acad. Sci. U.S.A.* **50**, 576.

LEWIS, W. H. & WRIGHT, E. S. (1935) On the development of the mouse. *Contr. Embryol.* **25**, 113.

MINTZ, B. (1962) Experimental study of the developing mammalian egg: removal of the zona pellucida. *Science, N.Y.* **138**, 594.

REPKE, K. (1964) Uber den biochemischen Wirkungsmodus von Digitalis. *Klin. Wschr.* **42**, 157.

SHAPIRO, H. (1941) Centrifugal elongation of cells, and some conditions governing the return to sphericity, and cleavage time. *J. cell. comp. Physiol.* **18**, 61.

SMITH, L. J. (1956) A morphological and histochemical investigation of a pre-implantation lethal (t^{12}) in the house mouse. *J. exp. Zool.* **132**, 51.

THOMSON, J. L. & BIGGERS, J. D. (1966) Effect of inhibitors of protein synthesis on the development of preimplantation mouse embryos. *Expl Cell Res.* **41**, 411.

VISHWAKARMA, P. & MILLER, T. (1963) Renal tubular transport of citrate: relations with calcium. *Am. J. Physiol.* **205**, 281.

WALES, R. G. & O'SHEA, T. (1966) The oxidative utilization of fructose and acetate by washed ram spermatozoa in the presence or absence of potassium and magnesium. *Aust. J. biol. Sci.* **19**, 167.

WHITTEN, W. K. (1957) Culture of tubal ova. *Nature, Lond.* **179**, 1081.

WHITTINGHAM, D. G. & BIGGERS, J. D. (1967) Fallopian tube and early cleavage in the mouse. *Nature, Lond.* **213**, 942.

157

Glycogen Content of Preimplantation Mouse Embryos

JOAN L. THOMSON AND RALPH L. BRINSTER

The energy metabolism of preimplantation mouse embryos has been investigated recently through *in vitro* culturing techniques (Brinster, '65a; Brinster and Thomson, '66). These experiments have led to a number of interesting observations regarding the energy requirements of the early embryo. First, cleavage of the one-cell mouse zygote will not occur completely *in vitro* (Biggers, Gwatkin and Brinster, '62); second, two-cell mouse embryos will develop into blastocysts *in vitro* in a medium containing pyruvate or lactate, but not glucose, as the only energy source (Brinster, '65a); third, eight-cell embryos will form blastocysts *in vitro* with pyruvate, lactate or glucose as the only source of energy (Brinster and Thomson, '66).

The possibility that an endogenous energy supply might exist in and be ulitized by the early mouse embryo led to the present investigation of glycogen content at various stages of development. Fridhandler ('61) has suggested that a stored energy source might be used by the early rabbit embryo. Earlier histochemical studies of ovarian sections of the rat (Wislocki, Bunting and Dempsey, '47; Harter, '48; Deane, '52), mouse (Goldman, '12), and cow (Kenney, '64) have shown that glycogen is present in the cytoplasm of ovarian ova. Lowenstein and Cohen ('64) have suggested that the one-cell mouse ovum contains approximately 16% of a carbohydrate material.

If it could be shown that the mouse embryo utilizes stored glycogen at some time during early development, some of the questions concerning the *in vitro* nutrient requirements might be more easily answered.

MATERIALS AND METHODS

Collection of embryos. Embryos were obtained from eight-week-old Swiss female mice, which were hormonally superovulated and mated with Swiss males. The embryos were collected by removing the fallopian tube, for early stages, or the tube plus uterus for later stages, and flushing out the tract with culture medium (Brinster, '63). On the first day after mating, embryos are one-cell and are still surrounded by cumulus cells. Some of these ova were treated with hyaluronidase to remove the cumulus mass and others were stained with these cells still attached. On the second day, embryos are two-cell; on the third day, mainly eight-cell; on the fourth day, morulae and early blastocysts;

and on the fifth day, late blastocysts which have emerged or hatched from the zona pellucida. Embryos collected at the two-cell stage and cultured *in vitro* follow the same developmental schedule (Brinster, '63).

Histological methods. Six to ten embryos of one stage were transferred to the center of a glass microscope slide with a minimum of culture medium. Initial fixation was carried out by exposing the embryos to an atmosphere of formalin and acetic acid vapor. The chambers used for this procedure were large petri dishes, containing gauze saturated with concentrated formalin and glacial acetic acid in a ratio of 1:1, and glass supports for the slides. After five to ten minutes, slides were removed from the chamber, and were slowly flooded with Tellyesniczky's fixative:

100% formalin	10 ml
glacial acetic acid	10 ml
95% ethanol	150 ml
distilled water	50 ml

The embryos were fixed for 15 to 20 minutes, then the slides were drained and stored in 70% alcohol in the refrigerator until fixation. This procedure serves not only to fix the embryos, but causes them to adhere to the slides, and removes the zonae pellucidae, which are soluble in acid.

Before staining, half of the slides of each stage were treated with 0.5% diastase at 37°C for two hours, in order to remove the glycogen. Control slides were incubated in distilled water under the same conditions. After thorough washing, the slides were placed in 0.5% periodic acid for ten minutes, then were washed again in running tap water. The embryos were stained for 15 minutes in Schiff's reagent, and were rinsed for two minutes in each of three changes of 0.5% $Na_2S_2O_5$. The slides were washed, dehydrated, and mounted in balsam. Areas of the embryos which were stained red in the controls, but not in the enzyme-treated embryos, were presumed to contain glycogen.

RESULTS

PAS-positive material is present in all stages of preimplantation mouse embryos (see figures), and no differences were found between embryos which had developed *in vivo* and those which were cultured *in vitro*. Control slides, treated with diastase before staining, were devoid of color for all stages, indicating that the PAS-positive material is glycogen.

The strongest positive reaction was found for two-cell, eight-cell and morula stages, where all blastomeres were stained a deep pink (figs. 2–4). Fertilized and unfertilized single-cell ova consistently appeared to be lighter in color, whether or not they were treated with hyaluronidase (fig. 1). In examining blastocysts at various stages of expansion, from the beginning of cavitation (fig. 5) to a late post-hatching stage (fig. 8), a decrease in the total amount of glycogen was found. The decrease was most obvious in the trophoblast cells, and glycogen was found, even in the latest stage, in the inner cell mass, although in very small quantities.

When embryos are cultured *in vitro* from the two-cell stage, there are always some which either fail to cleave at all, or which are arrested after one or more cleavages. Although some of these arrested embryos degenerate after three days in culture, many remain macroscopically normal. In studying the glycogen content of these arrested, but macroscopically normal, embryos, it was found that they retained their store of PAS-positive material in spite of their failure to develop.

DISCUSSION

One of the unexpected findings in this investigation was the apparent increase in glycogen content between the one-cell and the two-cell stage. Whether or not this change represents an actual increase in total glycogen content cannot be determined by this method. A possible explanation is the fact that there is a decrease in total volume of the embryo, from the one-cell to the two-cell stage, of approximately 18%. This decrease in volume would increase the concentration of glycogen and would result in a more intense staining in the two-cell embryo.

The fact that there was no decrease in glycogen from the two-cell stage to the morula was also surprising. Even though glucose can be used by the stages after the eight-cell, these stages did not utilize the glycogen which was present. In fact, only after blastocyst formation did the

PLATE 1

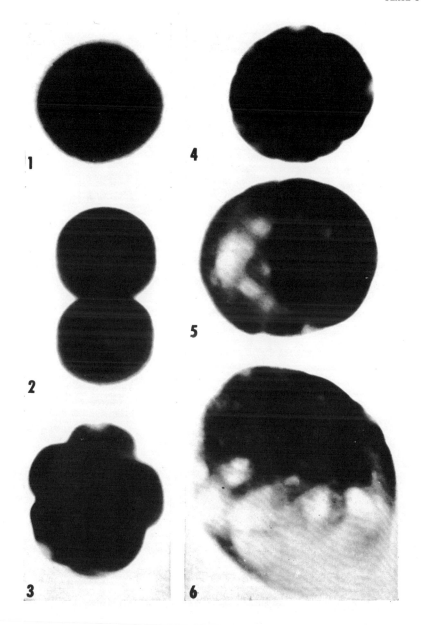

1

4

2

5

3

6

PLATE 2

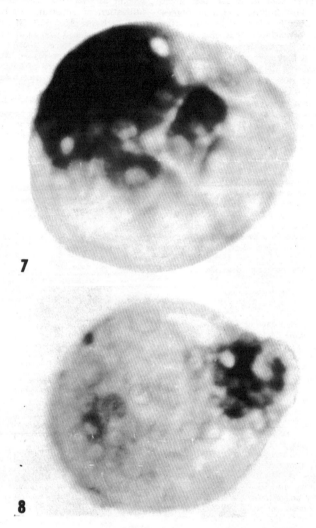

EXPLANATION OF FIGURES

Both figures are whole mounts of embryos which developed *in vivo*, stained by the periodic acid-Schiff method. × 340.

7 Blastocyst obtained four days after fertilization, showing positive material confined to the inner cell mass.

8 Late blastocyst obtained after hatching, on the fifth day after mating.

ovum appear able to utilize the stored glycogen. This finding seems to suggest that phosphorylase is active only after blastocyst formation. That this store is not available for use is further substantiated by the fact that ova grown *in vitro* did not show a decreased color reaction, even though one might expect the conditions *in vitro* to be nutritionally less adequate, so that the ova might rely more on endogenous stores.

Further studies (to be reported elsewhere) using the phosphorylase inhibitor phloridzin, indicated that blockage of the phosphorylase enzyme was without effect on *in vitro* development. Concentrations of phloridzin up to 10^{-3} M did not significantly affect development of the two-cell ova into blastocysts. This implies that phosphorylase activity is not essential for the development of these stages. Even the early blastocyst, in which a slight decrease in glycogen has been shown, was able to expand in the presence of the inhibitor. This evidence suggests that the glycogen present does not play an essential role in energy metabolism of the embryo at least up to the blastocyst stage (the fourth day of development).

The rapid decrease of PAS-positive, diastase-removable color in the blastocyst stages, first in the trophoblast and slightly later in the inner cell mass, seems to indicate that glycogen may be an important energy source during the fifth day of development, that is during expansion and hatching of the blastocyst. Exactly why the glycogen becomes available at this time is not definitely known but it seems probable that there are dramatic changes in the energy metabolism of the embryo during the cleavage stages. This is evidenced by the changes in the culture requirements of the mouse embryo mentioned above, and also by changes in enzyme activities during the first five days of development. Brinster ('65b) has shown that the lactic dehydrogenase activity of the mouse embryo is extremely high during the first three days of development, but that there is a seven-fold decrease in activity from the eight-cell stage to the blastocyst. This may indicate a sharp decrease in the embryo's dependency on exogenous lactate at this time and an increase in utilization of substrates such as glucose and perhaps glycogen. It would not be surprising to find that other enzymes, perhaps phosphorylase, change in activity during the cleavage stages. Such changes are probably evidence of basic changes in the pattern of energy metabolism.

ACKNOWLEDGMENTS

This investigation was supported in part by a Public Health Service post-doctoral fellowship HD-22,243-02 to Joan L. Thomson, from the Institute of Child Health and Human Development, and by a grant from the Population Council.

LITERATURE CITED

Biggers, J. D., R. B. L. Gwatkin and R. L. Brinster 1962 Development of mouse embryos in organ cultures of fallopian tubes on a chemically defined medium. Nature, *194:* 747–749.

Brinster, R. L. 1963 A method for *in vitro* cultivation of mouse ova from two-cell to blastocyst. Exp. Cell Res., *32:* 205–208.

——— 1965a Studies on the development of mouse embryos *in vitro*. II. The effect of energy source. J. Exp. Zool., *158:* 59–68.

——— 1965b Lactic dehydrogenase activity in the preimplanted mouse embryo. Biochim. Biophys. Acta, *110:* 439–441.

Brinster, R. L., and J. L. Thomson 1966 Development of eight-cell mouse embryos *in vitro*. Exp. Cell Res., *42:* 308–315.

Deane, H. 1952 Histochemical observations on the ovary and oviduct of the albino rat during the estrous cycle. Am. J. Anat., *91:* 363–413.

Fridhandler, L. 1961 Pathways of glucose metabolism in fertilized rabbit ova at various pre-implantation stages. Exp. Cell Res., *22:* 303–316.

Goldman, E. E. 1912 Neue Untersuchungen uber die äussere und innere Sekretion des gesunden organismus im Uchte der "vitalen Färbung." Teil 2. Beitrag. z. Klin. Chir., *78:* 1–108.

Harter, B. 1948 Glycogen and carbohydrate-protein complexes in the ovary of the white rat during the estrous cycle. Anat. Rec., *102:* 349–367.

Kenney, R. 1964 Histochemical and biochemical correlates of the estrus cycle in the normal cyclic uterus and ovary of the cow. Ph.D. Thesis, Cornell University.

Lowenstein, J. E., and A. I. Cohen 1964 Dry mass, lipid content and protein content of the intact and zona-free mouse ovum. J. Emb. Exp. Morph., *12:* 113–121.

Wislocki, G., H. Bunting and E. Dempsey 1947 Metachromasia in mammalian tissues and its relationship to mucopolysaccharides. Am. J. Anat., *81:* 1–38.

LACTATE DEHYDROGENASE ISOZYMES IN
MOUSE BLASTOCYST CULTURES

SUSAN AUERBACH and R. L. BRINSTER

Two types of peptide subunits, designated A and B, combine in all possible groups of four to form the usual 5 tetramers of lactate dehydrogenase (LDH) [1]. The five isozymes separable by electrophoresis are numbered from the most anodal form as follows: LDH-1 or B_4, LDH-2 or A_1B_3, LDH-3 or A_2B_2, LDH-4 or A_3B_1 and LDH-5 or A_4. The electrophoretic pattern of these forms reflects the proportion of the two types of subunit present in a sample and is characteristic for a given type of tissue, as well as for a given stage of development [10, 13]. We have previously found that the lactate dehydrogenase of preimplantation mouse embryos, from one-cell through blastocyst stages, consists of the most anodal isozyme, LDH-1. There is a drastic change to a predominance of isozyme LDH-5 associated with the process of implantation in the uterus, whether this occurs at the usual time on day 5 of pregnancy or at a later time when implantation is artificially delayed [2].

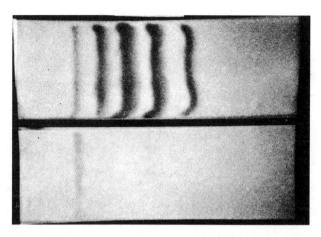

Fig. 1.—The top strip is mouse heart homogenate. The bottom strip is a sample of outgrowths from 150 blastocysts. Electrophoretic migration is from the left edge of the strip toward the right (anode) and the corresponding bands of enzyme activity are LDH-5 (A_4), LDH-4 (A_3B), LDH-3 (A_2B_2), LDH-2 (AB_3), and LDH-1 (B_4).

It has been found [6, 9, 11] that when mouse blastocysts are placed in culture medium containing serum, there is an attachment of the blastocysts to the culture dish, with a subsequent flattening and proliferation of the cells. We now find that this change in morphology of the blastocyst *in vitro* also is associated with changes in LDH isozyme pattern.

Blastocysts were obtained in two ways. Some were collected by flushing the uteri of day-4 pregnant Swiss mice, as described by Brinster [3]. For most experiments, blastocysts were obtained from mouse embryo cultures which had been grown from the two-cell stage *in vitro* for three days in medium BMOC-2 [4]. The blastocysts collected in either of these two ways were placed in plastic culture dishes in drops of medium under paraffin oil [3]. The medium used for blastocyst outgrowth was Eagle's medium, BME diploid with glutamine [7], supplemented with 1 per cent to 5 per cent fetal calf serum (Grand Island Biological Co., Grand Island, N.Y.) [9] and 100 units/l penicillin G plus 50 μg/l streptomycin sulfate [4]. After 4 days in culture, the blastocysts had attached to the dish, flattened and grown outward. Groups of these outgrowths were collected in a few microliters of medium and frozen at $-70°C$. The LDH was liberated into the solution by subsequent thawing, and these samples were subjected to cellulose acetate electrophoresis for LDH isozymes [2], or assay for LDH activity [5] in a Beckman DU spectrophotometer adapted with microcells [8]

Fig. 1 shows that the LDH of the blastocyst outgrowths migrates as isozyme 5. Equal aliquots of the medium alone gave no LDH bands. In order to eliminate the possibility that the change in isozyme pattern was due to a degeneration of the LDH-1 with a very small percentage of LDH-5 remaining and made apparent by use of a larger amount of tissue for electrophoresis, the total amount of LDH activity per embryo was measured. In each of three experiments, eight groups of 10 to 15 outgrowths were assayed for total activity. The mean values with the standard errors were $0.31 \pm 0.03 \times 10^{-8}$ moles, $0.32 \pm 0.02 \times 10^{-8}$ moles, and $0.25 \pm 0.01 \times 10^{-8}$ moles of reduced nicotinamide adenine dinucleotide ($NADH_2$) oxidized per h per outgrowth. In comparison, late blastocysts before culturing have the isozyme LDH-1 [2, 12] with a total activity of $0.51 \pm 0.04 \times 10^{-8}$ moles NADH oxidized per h per blastocyst [5]. This similarity of levels of LDH activity between the day 5 blastocyst and the blastocyst outgrowths, in conjunction with the dramatic change in isozyme pattern from type 1 to type 5 respectively, indicates that the culture conditions which induce the attachment and outgrowth of the blastocyst also induce the synthesis of the A type peptide subunits of the enzyme.

This synthesis of A type subunits of LDH and the coincident change in pattern from type 1 to type 5 isozyme has now been shown to occur in the early mouse embryo under two conditions. The first is when the embryo implants normally in the uterus of the mouse [2], and the second is when the embryo attaches to the culture surface as described above. Early cleavage stage embryos cannot be induced to change isozyme pattern from LDH-1 to LDH-5 when they are cultured to the blastocyst stage in the same type of medium which induces the characteristic blastocyst attachment. It appears that the embryo may be resistant to the "induction" of the pa tern change until a certain morphological or developmental stage is reached. After this critical stage is attained, more than one stimulus may be able to initiate synthesis of the type A peptide subunits. Whether the *in vitro* attachment of the embryo to the culture surface simulates the *in vivo* attachment of the embryo to the uterus in respect to initiating type A peptide synthesis, or whether the synthesis is brought about by a general differentiation of cells in culture is not known. Further work is in progress to answer this question.

Summary.—When mouse blastocysts are cultured in Eagle's medium plus serum, which promotes attachment to the dish and proliferation of the cells, their lactate dehydrogenase isozyme electrophoresis pattern changes from LDH-1 to LDH-5.

This work was supported by grant HD-00239 from the National Institutes of Health and was done during the tenure by one of us (S. A.) of a US Public Health Service predoctoral fellowship (training grant GM-00694-07).

REFERENCES

1. APPELLA, E. and MARKERT, C. L., *Biochem. Biophys. Res. Comm.* **6**, 171 (1961).
2. AUERBACH, S. and BRINSTER, R. L., *Exptl Cell Res.* **46**, 89 (1967).
3. BRINSTER, R. L., *Exptl Cell Res.* **32**, 205 (1963)
4. —— *J. Reprod. Fertil.* **10**, 227 (1965).
5. —— *Biochim. Biophys. Acta* **110**, 439 (1965).
6. COLE, R. V. and PAUL, J., *in* WOLSTENHOLME, G. E. W. and O'CONNOR, M. (eds), Preimplantation Stages of Pregnancy, p. 82. Little, Brown and Co, Boston, 1965.
7. EAGLE, H., *Science* **122**, 501 (1955).
8. GREENBERG, L. J. and RODDER, J. A., *Analyt. Biochem.* **8**, 137 (1964).
9. GWATKIN, R. B. L., *Ann. N.Y. Acad. Sci.* **139**, 79 (1966).
10. MARKERT, C. L. and MOLLER, F., *Proc. Natl Acad. Sci. US* **45**, 753 (1959).
11. MINTZ, B., *J. Exptl Zool.* **157**, 273 (1964).
12. RAPOLA, J. and KOSKIMIES, O., *Science* **157**, 1311 (1967).
13. WIELAND, T. and PFLEIDERER, G., *Biochem. Z.* **329**, 112 (1957).

LACTATE DEHYDROGENASE ISOZYMES IN THE
EARLY MOUSE EMBRYO

SUSAN AUERBACH and R. L. BRINSTER

THE unusually high specific activity of lactate dehydrogenase (LDH) in the mouse embryo [5] and the ability of the two-cell mouse ovum to use lactate as its only energy source [3] suggested the importance of LDH to the early developmental stages. An examination of the isozyme pattern of the embryo has shown a shift from type 1 (B subunits) during the first five days of development to type 5 (A subunits) after implantation of the embryo. The possibility of gaining insight into the metabolism of the early mouse embryo, and of using an *in vitro* system [2] for investigating the mechanism of regulation of protein synthesis in the early mammalian embryo has led to the study described here.

The isozymes of LDH have been investigated in the tissues of many animals. Two subunit types make up the usual five tetramers separable by electrophoresis, these have different kinetic properties and are thought to have different metabolic roles [1, 6, 8, 14, 15]. Activity patterns, representing the relative abundance of the two types, are characteristic of particular kinds of tissues, and are constant and characteristic of the particular stage of development. Studies with the deer mouse have shown the two subunits to be under separate genetic control [13], and therefore ontogeny of the enzyme pattern is presumably the result of differential gene expression.

Markert and Ursprung [9] described the ontogeny of LDH patterns in mouse tissues from the 12 day fetus to the adult. They found that for all embryonic tissues the LDH-5 band was the principal type. After day 12 of development there was a gradual shift in some tissues toward predominance of the anodic type. The apparent one way shift toward the LDH-1 form with age led them to extrapolate and conclude that the "embryonic form" of LDH in the mouse was LDH-5. Hinks and Masters [7] followed the pattern ontogeny in the rabbit from the 10-day fetus to the adult. They found that in skeletal muscle the percent of LDH-1 gradually increases during fetal development, then decreases just before birth and continues to decrease after birth. On the basis of their experiments, they suggested abandoning the "embryonic form" information obtained from half-grown fetuses.

MATERIALS AND METHODS

In our experiments, zone electrophoresis of homogenates was done on cellulose acetate strips in tris-barbital buffer pH 8.8, ionic strength 0.025, 31 volts/cm at 4°C for 75 min. To localize the enzyme bands, each cellulose acetate strip was covered with another strip previously dipped in the following reagent mixture: 2 ml of 1 M sodium lactate, 6 ml of 1 mg/ml nitroblue tetrazolium, 0.6 ml of 1 mg/ml phenazine methosulfate, 2 ml tris-barbital buffer pH 8.8 ionic strength 0.05, and 20 mg NAD.[1] Ova were collected from superovulated, random bred Swiss mice by the methods described by Brinster [2].

RESULTS

The strips were incubated in the dark for 30 min. Samples of unfertilized ova, one-cell ova, two-cell ova, blastocysts removed from the uterus on the fifth day of pregnancy, and two-cell ova grown *in vitro* to blastocysts for three days, all showed an isozyme pattern characterized by predominantly type 1 LDH. In contrast, samples from fetuses of 7 through 12 days gestation (implanted embryos) gave patterns with a large proportion of LDH-5. Fig. 1 is a typical zymogram. The samples from adult heart and skeletal muscle were reference markers for migration distance. The samples of unfertilized ova, 9-day fetuses, and 9-day decidua (uterus) tissue were run at approximately equal activities (4.7 μmoles NADH$_2$ oxidized in 10 min by 10^{-3} M pyruvate at 37°C, pH 7.5, approximately equal to the LDH activity in 60 one-cell ova) to demonstrate the differences in relative abundance of the two types of subunits. The distribution of the 2 subunits (A and B) among tetramers of LDH in a single tissue usually follows the binomial distribution to the fourth power. Band intensity ratios give a rough approximation of the amount of each subunit present. From Fig. 1 there appears to be over 98 per cent B subunit in the unfertilized ova and approximately 90 per cent A subunit in the 9-day fetus. On the ninth day, the total amount of LDH activity per embryo is approximately fifty times that of the one-cell egg. Thus by day 9 the embryo has synthesized a considerable amount of the A subunit. The activity in 8-day embryos and 7-day embryos is predominantly LDH-5. The data indicate an extreme shift in the proportion of the two subunits in the embryo some time between the fifth day and the seventh day of pregnancy. Implantation occurs on the sixth day.

---

[1] Apparatus and method from Gelman Instrument Co., Ann Arbor, Michigan.

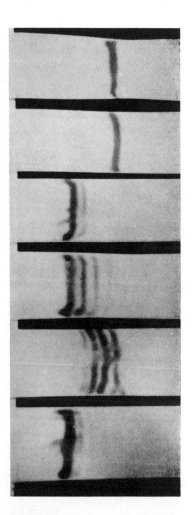

Fig. 1.—From top to bottom, the first two strips are samples of one-cell ova, third strip nine-day fetus, fourth strip nine-day decidua, fifth strip adult heart, sixth strip adult skeletal muscle. The start is marked by the edge of the black paper and migration is toward the right (anode). The first four strips were run at equal total LDH activities. From left to right the bands represent LDH-5 (A_4), LDH-4 (A_3B), LDH-3 (A_2B_2), LDH-2 (AB_3), and LDH-1 (B_4).

That the isozyme change is associated with the actual process of implantation was shown by an examination of older, yet viable, blastocysts. In natural postpartum pregnancy, or in mice ovariectomized on the 3rd day of pregnancy, with pregnancy maintained by injection of 1 mg of progesterone/mouse/day, the blastocysts form in the usual time but remain unattached in the uterus for a longer time [11]. When lactation stops or estrogen is injected, the blastocysts implant and the remainder of gestation is normal. Blastocysts flushed from the uterine lumens of ovariectomized mice on the eighth day of pregnancy also show the LDH-1 band; their gross morphology is the same as that of normal 5 day blastocysts rather than that of 8-day embryos. This strongly suggests that the mechanism responsible for the initiation of the synthesis of A type subunits is related to implantation and not to the time elapsed since fertilization.

DISCUSSION

In view of the small amount of available information concerning the metabolism of the early mouse embryo, the role of the enzyme still must be speculative [4]. However, the concentration of lactate in the fallopian tube during the first three days of pregnancy in the rabbit [10] is between 0.8×10^{-3} M and 5.7×10^{-3} M. Determination of K_m observed for lactate [12] are 9×10^{-3} M for beef LDH-1 and 7×10^{-3} M for chicken LDH-1 as opposed to 2.5×10^{-2} M for beef LDH and 4×10^{-2} M for chicken LDH-5. It is tempting to speculate that the zygote has both a high LDH content and predominantly LDH type 1 in order to efficiently utilize the concentration of lactate found in the fallopian tube [12].

SUMMARY

The lactate dehydrogenase of the cleavage and blastocyst stages of the mouse embryo is predominantly the LDH-1 type. A change to predominantly LDH-5 is associated with the process of implantation into the uterus.

We are indebted to the Population Council, Inc. (M-65), the National Science Foundation (GB 4465), and the National Institutes of Health (5-TI-GM-694-05) for financial support.

REFERENCES

1. APPELLA, E. and MARKERT, C. L., *Biochem. Biophys. Res. Comm.* 6, 171 (1961).
2. BRINSTER, R. L., *Exptl Cell Res.* 32, 205 (1963).
3. —— *J. Exptl Zool.* 158, 59 (1965).
4. —— in G. E. W. WOLSTENHOLME and M. O'CONNER (eds.), Preimplantation stages of pregnancy, p. 60. Little, Brown and Co., Boston, 1965.
5. —— *Biochim. Biophys. Acta* 110, 439 (1965).
6. DAWSON, D. M., GOODFRIEND, T. L. and KAPLAN, N. O., *Science* 143, 929 (1964).
7. HINKS, M. and MASTERS, C. J., *Life Sci.* 4, 697 (1965).
8. KAPLAN, N. O., *Brookhaven Symp. Biol.* 17, 131 (1964).
9. MARKERT, C. L. and URSPRUNG, H., *Devel. Biol.* 5, 363 (1962).
10. MASTROIANNI, L. JR. and WALLACH, R. C., *Am. J. Physiol.* 200, 815 (1961).
11. MAYER, G., in A. C. ENDERS (ed.), Delayed implantation, p. 213. Univ. of Chicago Press, Chicago, 1963.
12. PESCE, A., McKAY, R. H., STOLZENBACH, F., CAHN, R. D. and KAPLAN, N. O., *J. Biol. Chem.* 239, 1753 (1964).
13. SHAW, C. R. and BARTO, E., *Proc. Natl Acad Sci. U.S.* 50, 211 (1963).
14. STAMBAUGH, R. and POST, D., *J. Biol. Chem.* 241, 1462 (1966).
15. WIELAND, T. and PFLIEDERER, G., *Angew. Chem. Internat. Ed. (English)* 1, 169 (1962).

THE PATTERN OF UTILIZATION OF RESPIRATORY
METABOLIC INTERMEDIATES BY PREIMPLANTATION RABBIT
EMBRYOS *IN VITRO*

J. C. DANIEL, Jr.

The pathways of glucose metabolism obviously change during early development of mammal embryos. Presumably these changes are reflections of a "lack of necessary enzyme systems" [5] in early stages and the subsequent "...emergence of an enzyme

171

complex during development" [12]. The purpose of the studies reported in this paper has been to define the time and sequence of onset of respiratory pathways by determining which metabolic intermediates could be utilized as energy sources for growth by different age rabbit embryos *in vitro*.

Methods and Materials.—The general methods of growing rabbit embryos *in vitro* have been described in earlier publications [7–10]. For the present work the method was essentially as follows:

Rabbit embryos of ages one through seven days *post coitum* were removed from the genital tract by either flushing or being lifted from the endometrial surface of an opened uterus, whichever method best fit the particular embryo in question. The embryos were rinsed twice in F10 medium [13] without glucose or pyruvate and then retained in plastic organ culture dishes, in 1 cc of F10 medium, devoid of all but one energy source. For the early ages (cleavage stages) the number of cells, and for the later ages (blastocysts) the diameters, were recorded at the beginning of each experiment and again 12 and 24 hr later. Thus the utilization of a given substance was expressed as its ability to support growth over these periods. From 5 to 7 specimens taken from at least two different mothers were used at each age for each substance tested. The concentration of 5×10^{-3} M, except in a few cases where the large size of the molecule made it impractical, was selected as comparable to concentrations of glucose, pyruvate and lactate determined earlier as favorable to the growth of 5-day blastocysts *in vitro* [9]. When this concentration was obviously toxic, as with D-glyceraldehyde-3-phosphate or with D-glyceraldehyde, the experiments were repeated at a 1/10 dilution.

Results.—Fig. 1 demonstrates graphically the results obtained.

Some variation in the embryonic stages occurred even though they were removed as promptly at 24 hr intervals after breeding, as the manipulations would permit. One-day ova were mostly at the 2-cell stage with less than 10 per cent at 1- or 4-cell stages, 2-day ones were typically at 16 cells, and 3-day at mid-morula. At the 4-day period about half of the embryos were early blastocysts and the remaining half were late morulae. Days 5, 6 and 7 were successively more advanced blastocysts with embryonic discs obvious on day 6 and embryonic shields forming by day 7.

The results might be summarized as follows:

Stage	1st utilization of substrate for 24 hr of growth
2 cells	Phosphoenol pyruvate, pyruvate, lactate
16 cells	6-phosphogluconate
Mid-morula	Acetate (?)
Late morula	*Cis*-aconitate, α-Ketoglutarate, α-D-glucose-1-phosphate (?)
Early-blastocyst	Glucose, D-galactose, glycogen, D-glucose-6-phosphate, Fumarate, oxaloacetate (?), succinate, malate (?)
Mid-blastocyst	D-fructose
	D-isocitrate
Late-blastocyst	D-fructose-1, 6-diphosphate
	Acetyl coenzyme A, citrate

When D-glyceraldehyde and D-glyceraldehyde-3-phosphate were used at the 5×10^{-3} M concentration, all the embryos of all stages tested were darkened and

	1 day	2 days	3 days	4 days	5 days	6 days	7 days	Concentration
D-Glucose								$5 \times 10^{-3} M$
D-Glucose-6-phosphate								$5 \times 10^{-3} M$
D-Fructose-1, 6-diphosphate								$5 \times 10^{-3} M$
D-Glyceraldehyde-3-phosphate								$5 \times 10^{-3} M$
Phospho-enolpyruvate								$5 \times 10^{-3} M$
Pyruvate								$5 \times 10^{-3} M$
Acetyl coenzyme A								$5 \times 10^{-4} M$
Citrate								$5 \times 10^{-3} M$
Cis-aconitate								$5 \times 10^{-3} M$
D-Isocitrate								$5 \times 10^{-3} M$
α-Ketoglutarate								$5 \times 10^{-3} M$
Succinate								$5 \times 10^{-3} M$
Fumarate								$5 \times 10^{-3} M$
Malate								$5 \times 10^{-3} M$
Oxaloacetate								$5 \times 10^{-3} M$
Glycogen								$5 \times 10^{-7} M$
α-D-Glucose-1-phosphate								$5 \times 10^{-3} M$
D-Galactose								$5 \times 10^{-3} M$
D-Fructose								$5 \times 10^{-3} M$
D-Glyceraldehyde								$5 \times 10^{-3} M$
L-Lactate								$5 \times 10^{-3} M$
Acetate								$5 \times 10^{-3} M$
6-Phosphogluconate								$5 \times 10^{-3} M$
Full medium								
Metabolite-free medium								

Fig. 1.—Growth *in vitro* of rabbit embryos of ages 1 through 7 days *post coitum*, with various energy sources. Each circle is a separate embryo; open if there was no growth, solid if growth continued for 24 hr, half-open if some growth was observed by 12 hr but did not continue for 24 hr.

collapsed by the 12 hr observation. When these same intermediates were tested at a lower concentration ($5 \times 10^{-4} M$) the embryos appeared normal and viable but in no case was any growth observed.

Discussion.—It is apparent, after reference to Fig. 1, that the first consistent utilization of most of the intermediates tested is by blastocyst stages. The occasional specimen from the early cleavage stages (day 1 and 2) that showed some growth by 12 hr, had merely completed a cleavage that was probably imminent at the time the experiment was initiated. It has been difficult to get good growth *in vitro* of mammal blastocysts at the early blastocyst stage [19], so days 3 and 4 represent special problem areas. It will be noted that most of the specimens of these ages did not grow even in full medium. The full medium contains both pyruvate and glucose and since both 3- and 4-day stages grew in pyruvate alone, one is led to suspect some inhibition of growth of these stages by glucose.

173

The 5- and 6-day-old blastocysts gave the most consistent results in each experiment but some minimal growth of these stages was achieved even in the controls in metabolite-free medium, presumably as a result of some storage in the cells or in the relatively large amount of blastocyst fluid they contain. Growth of the 7-day stages was generally not as good as 5- and 6-day stages in the same medium (except glucose and galactose), possibly because of more rapid depletion of the available nutrients by a much larger embryo.

Some of the variability in the results is undoubtedly reflective of the variability of the specimens used at each stage. For example, the 4-day embryos that did not grow in D-glucose-6-phosphate were at the morula stage while the ones that showed growth were already blastocysts. And, the 5-day ones that grew were larger blastocysts than those that failed to grow. Similar results were observed with fumarate.

These data are consistent with, and lend further support to several earlier observations concerning the utilization of energy intermediates by early mammal embryos [4, 5, 11, 12, 14, 16, 17]. In this connection, it is of interest to point out certain similarities that exist between rabbit and mouse embryos. For instance, the growth of tubal mouse ova can be supported *in vitro* by lactate and pyruvate but not by acetate or citrate [22]. Brinster [4] reported that 2-cell mouse ova will grow to blastocysts in medium containing lactate, pyruvate, or phosphoenol pyruvate but not glucose, fructose, glucose-6-phosphate, fructose-1,6-phosphate, acetate, citrate, ketoglutarate, succinate, fumarate or malate.

Differences also exist; for example, the 2-cell mouse ovum will grow in oxalacetate [5] as distinct from rabbit ova. It is to be noted, however, that growth of all stages of the rabbit was poor in oxaloacetate, so these data may reflect another factor, possibly toxic concentration. Furthermore, the mouse ovum can utilize glucose by the 4-cell-stage [5], a capacity not existing in the rabbit embryo until the blastocyst (or possibly late morula) stage [11, 12].

Rabbit ova utilize oxygen [11, 12, 20] and are inhibited by anaerobic conditions and by cyanide [12, 17]. Contrary to this, the mouse embryo at the tubal ovum stage [22], and the blastocyst stage [18], and the pre- and early-somite rat embryo [1] all continue to grow in an anaerobic environment.

Evidence has been obtained for the presence of certain key respiratory enzymes in early mammal embryos [3, 6, 15] and one might attempt to interpret the differences in utilization of oxygen or energy intermediates by different embryos, in the light of the activities of these enzymes.

Pyruvate, phosphoenolpyruvate, and lactate seem to be the only substrates that can support growth of initial cleavage stages. That 6-phosphogluconate does not support growth until the second day, is evidence that the pentose shunt may not be utilized by the single- and 2-cell stages.

In view of the need for pyruvate (or similar substance) by the early rabbit embryo and its apparent oxygen requirement, one seems forced to the conclusion that the citric acid cycle is functioning, perhaps at the minimal level, but can only be entered as pyruvate. The pentose shunt may be functional by the 8–16-cell stage and the Embden-Meyerhof pathway functional by the blastocyst stage. It is difficult to infer from these data that any period exists when the pre-implantation rabbit embryo is dependent entirely on anaerobic glycolysis.

The experiments reported here do not rule out the possibility that pyruvate might be required by these embryos for some reason other than its role in respiration, for example in the synthesis of fatty acids, steroids, neuraminic acids or some amino acids. If this were true, in view of the failure of 1-day embryos to grow in anything except pyruvate or substances closely related to it, then the true energy sources for these very early cleavage stages would most likely be in intercellular stores [12], or possibly in secreted coatings such as the mucin layer from the oviduct or the gloiolemma deposited around the blastocyst in the uterus [2]. Whittingham [23] has recently postulated an exogenous energy source in the mouse, secreted by the Fallopian tube and necessary for cleavage to occur.

The question of transport is important here and has been discussed [5]. The work of Wales and Biggers [21] "suggests that there is little or no uptake of malate by 2-cell mouse embryos and that an active uptake occurs by the 8-cell stage". However, the differences observed in uptake may in part reflect the observation of the same authors that the 8-cell stage is *utilizing* malate as a substrate while the 2-cell stage ovum is not. Nevertheless, the fact remains that glucose, which has no trouble traversing cell membranes, does not support growth until the blastocyst stage, a time coincidental with that when most of the intermediates do likewise.

Summary.—Rabbit embryos, recovered from the mother on any of days 1 through 7 *post coitum*, were cultured in different media containing a single respiratory metabolic intermediate. Their ability to grow *in vitro* for 12 or 24 hr was considered evidence that they were utilizing the particular energy source. Most of the intermediates will support growth of blastocysts but the initial cleavage stages will only grow in the presence of pyruvate, phosphoenol pyruvate, or lactate. From these results it is concluded that the citric acid cycle is functional in the earliest stages but that the Embden–Meyerhof pathway does not appear until several days later. The pentose shunt might be utilized by day-2 ova but not earlier ones.

The research was supported by N.S. F. Grant No. G.B. 4401.
The author is grateful to Dr R. S. Krishnan for his constructive criticism.

REFERENCES

1. BOELL, E. J., in WILLIER, WEISS and HAMBURGER (eds.), Analysis of Development, p. 520, 1955.
2. BOVING, B. G., *Cold Spring Harbor Symposia Quant. Biol.* **19**, 9 (1954).
3. BRINSTER, R. L., *Biochim. Biophys. Acta* **110**, 439 (1965).
4. —— *J. Exptl Zool.* **158**, 59 (1965).
5. —— *J. Reprod. Fertil.* **10**, 227 (1965).
6. —— *Exptl Cell Res.* **43**, 131 (1966).
7. DANIEL, J. C., *Am. Zool.* **3**, 526 (1963).
8. —— *Nature* **201**, 316 (1964).
9. —— *J. Embryol. Exptl Morphol.* **13**, 83 (1965).
10. —— *Third Teratology Workshop Supplement* (1966).
11. FRIDHANDLER, L., *Exptl Cell Res.* **22**, 303 (1961).
12. FRIDHANDLER, L., HAFEZ, E. S. E. and PINCUS, G., *Exptl Cell Res.* **13**, 132 (1957).
13. HAM, R. G., *Exptl Cell Res.* **29**, 515 (1963).
14. HUFF, R. L., EIK-NES, K. B., *J. Reprod. Fertil.* **11**, 57 (1966).
15. ISHIDA, K. and CHANG, M. C., *J. Histochem. Cytochem.* **13**, 470 (1965).
16. MOUNIB, M. S. and CHANG, M. C., *Exptl Cell Res.* **38**, 201 (1965).

17. PINCUS, G., *Science* **93**, 438 (1931).
18. POPP, R. A., *J. Exptl Zool.* **138**, 1 (1958).
19. PURSHOTTAM, N. and PINCUS, G., *Anat. Rec* **140**, 51 (1961).
20. SMITH, A. H. and KLEIBER, M., *J. Cell. Comp. Physiol.* **35**, 131 (1950).
21. WALES, R. G. and BIGGERS, J. D., *J. Cell Biol.* **31**, 120 A (1966).
22. WHITTEN, W. K., *Nature* **179**, 1081 (1957).
23. WHITTINGHAM, D. G., *J. Cell Biol.* **31**, 123 A (1966).

EFFECT OF NUCLEOSIDES AND NUCLEOSIDE BASES ON THE DEVELOPMENT OF PRE-IMPLANTATION MOUSE EMBRYOS *IN VITRO*

JOAN THOMSON TenBROECK

The nutritional requirements for the development *in vitro* of 2-celled mouse embryos into blastocysts have been extensively investigated by Brinster (1965a, b, c). It was found that most 2-celled embryos will develop normally in a culture medium consisting of bicarbonate-buffered Krebs-Ringer solution, containing bovine serum albumin as a protein source, and pyruvate and lactate as energy sources. Since there are always some 2-celled embryos which will not develop into blastocysts in this medium, the possibility exists that some other growth factors might increase the percentage of normally developing embryos. It is known that synthesis of DNA takes place throughout the cleavage stages and that RNA synthesis also occurs, especially after the 4-cell stage (Mintz, 1964). Thus it was thought that the addition of nucleic acid components to the culture medium might be beneficial for development.

Two-celled embryos for the experiments were collected from Swiss mice which had been superovulated and mated with Swiss males 2 days previously (Brinster, 1963). Embryos were cultured in small drops of medium under paraffin oil in 15 × 60 mm plastic tissue culture dishes. The cultures were maintained at 37° C in an atmosphere of humidified 5% CO_2 in air for 3 days, the time necessary for the formation of blastocysts from 2-celled embryos. To test single components, the compounds were added to culture medium at a concentration of 10^{-2} M, except for guanosine, which was insoluble above 10^{-3} M. In all cases the solutions were adjusted to maintain the optimum pH and osmolarity. To determine dose–response relationships for the compounds, a series of four tenfold dilutions was made from each of the initial solutions. Embryos were cultured in the various concentrations of the compounds for 3 days. In each case twelve embryos were placed in a drop, and two drops were allotted to each treatment. The entire series of experiments was repeated, so that a total of forty-eight embryos received each treatment. The experiments were scored by counting the number of morphologically normal blastocysts which developed in each drop. The fractional scores were converted to angles (Biggers & Brinster, 1965), and the data for each compound were subjected to an analysis of variance.

To test a combination of compounds, the bases adenine, cytosine, thymine and uracil were added to the culture medium, each at a concentration of 10^{-3} M;

177

guanine concentration was less than 10^{-3} M, because of the relative insolubility of this compound in aqueous solutions. Four ten-fold dilutions of this medium were made, and the effects of the various media on *in vitro* development were tested. The experimental design and analysis were identical with those of the single-component experiments. The effect of nucleoside combinations was tested

TABLE 1

EFFECT OF SOME PURINE AND PYRIMIDINE BASES ON THE DEVELOPMENT OF 2-CELL MOUSE EMBRYOS INTO BLASTOCYSTS *in vitro*

Treatment	Percentage of embryos forming blastocysts					
	0	$10^{-6}M$	$10^{-5}M$	$10^{-4}M$	$10^{-3}M$	$10^{-2}M$
Adenine	52·1	39·6	47·9	29·2	10·4	0
Cytosine	37·5	—	33·3	22·9	27·1	22·9
Thymine	62·5	66·7	45·8	54·2	56·2	2·08
Uracil	62·5	62·5	70·8	77·1	72·9	0

TABLE 2

EFFECT OF SOME NUCLEOSIDES ON THE DEVELOPMENT OF TWO-CELL MOUSE EMBRYOS INTO BLASTOCYSTS *in vitro*

Treatment	Percentage of embryos forming blastocysts					
	0	$10^{-6}M$	$10^{-5}M$	$10^{-4}M$	$10^{-3}M$	$10^{-2}M$
Adenosine	68·7	50·0	60·4	2·08	0	0
Cytidine	62·5	75·0	77·1	72·9	58·3	0
Guanosine	81·2	77·1	83·3	41·7	4·17	—
Thymidine	56·2	—	35·4	43·7	35·4	18·7
Uridine	39·6	—	20·8	35·4	10·4	2·08

TABLE 3

EFFECT OF BASE AND NUCLEOTIDE COMBINATIONS ON THE DEVELOPMENT OF 2-CELL MOUSE EMBRYOS INTO BLASTOCYSTS *in vitro*

Treatment	Percentage of embryos forming blastocysts					
	0	$10^{-7}M$	$10^{-6}M$	$10^{-5}M$	$10^{-4}M$	$10^{-3}M$
Bases	66·7	47·9	39·6	31·2	35·4	20·8
Nucleosides	66·7	56·2	47·9	52·1	16·7	2·08

by adding adenosine, cytidine, guanosine, thymidine and uridine to the medium, each at a concentration of 10^{-3} M. The medium was diluted and tested as previously described.

The results of the experiments with single bases and nucleosides are presented in Tables 1 and 2. Most of the compounds were increasingly inhibitory as the concentration was raised. The two main exceptions were cytidine and uracil, but, although the lower concentrations of both compounds resulted in an

178

increase in the number of blastocysts forming, these differences were not statistically significant.

The results of experiments using combinations of compounds are shown in Table 3. In the case of both nucleosides and bases, the compounds were increasingly inhibitory as the concentrations were increased.

The experiments have thus shown that the presence of nucleic acid precursors in the culture environment, either singly or in combination, does not enhance development of the pre-implantation mouse embryo. Since experiments with labelled nucleosides have shown that these compounds are incorporated by the early mouse embryo (Mintz, 1964; Monesi & Salfi, 1967), the lack of beneficial effect cannot be due to impermeability of the embryos to the compounds. It therefore appears likely that the early embryo either contains an adequate endogenous supply or is able to synthesize the components required for the formation of DNA and RNA.

This investigation was supported in part from a grant from the National Institutes of Health (HD-02315-02). The author acknowledges the excellent technical assistance of Miss Mary Ryans, Mrs Margaret van Meter and Miss Shelly Walker.

REFERENCES

BIGGERS, J. D. & BRINSTER, R. L. (1965) Biometrical problems in the study of early mammalian embryos *in vitro*. *J. exp. Zool.* **158,** 39.

BRINSTER, R. L. (1963) A method for *in vitro* cultivation of mouse ova from two-cell to blastocyst. *Expl Cell Res.* **32,** 205.

BRINSTER, R. L. (1965a) Studies on the development of mouse embryos *in vitro*. II. The effect of energy source. *J. exp. Zool.* **158,** 59.

BRINSTER, R. L. (1965b) Studies on the development of mouse embryos *in vitro*. III. The effect of fixed-nitrogen source. *J. exp. Zool.* **158,** 69.

BRINSTER, R. L. (1965c) Studies on the development of mouse embryos *in vitro*. IV. Interaction of energy sources. *J. Reprod. Fert.* **10,** 227.

MINTZ, B. (1964) Synthetic processes and early development in the mammalian egg. *J. exp. Zool.* **157,** 85.

MONESI, V. & SALFI, V. (1967) Macromolecular syntheses during early development in the mouse embryo. *Expl Cell Res.* **46,** 632.

Nucleic Acid Synthesis in Preimplantation Rabbit Embryos

I. QUANTITATIVE ASPECTS, RELATIONSHIP TO EARLY MORPHOGENESIS AND PROTEIN SYNTHESIS

COLE MANES

The molecular basis of embryogenesis in mammals has not been studied with the thoroughness which has characterized studies of echinoderm, amphibian, and avian systems, primarily because mammalian embryos are not normally available in large numbers. The use of hormonal superovulation has largely overcome this obstacle, and this technique, along with improvements in the *in vitro* maintenance of preimplantation embryos, has made possible the investigation of the very earliest syntheses carried on by the developing mammal. The work presented here concerns measurements of the rate of incorporation of uridine-H^3 by preimplantation rabbit embryos *in vitro* at daily intervals throughout the preimplantation period. These measurements are correlated with estimates of total embryonic ribonucleic acid as determined by the orcinol reaction.

Since embryogenesis is a matter of differential genetic expression, and since conversion of genetic information into cellular phenotype requires the synthesis of two distinct species of biopolymers, ribonucleic acids (RNA) and polypeptides, the present studies were undertaken with the intention of exploring genetic expression during preimplantation rabbit development at the level of RNA synthesis. The information reported here is compared with that previously obtained on protein synthesis during the same developmental period (Manes and Daniel, '69).

Considerable information has been published in the past few years regarding RNA and protein synthesis in preimplantation mouse embryos (Mintz, '64; Monesi and Salfi, '67; Ellem and Gwatkin, '68; Woodland and Graham, '69). Corresponding information from other mammalian orders, such as *Lagomorpha*, will supplement the studies of rodent embryogenesis in important ways. The rabbit ovum, for example, is about twice the diameter of the mouse ovum, cleaves more rapidly, reaches a morula stage of some 100–130 cells before cavitation begins, and retains it zona pellucida throughout the preimplantation period. For these reasons, it is perhaps not surprising that rabbit and mouse display differences in synthetic patterns. The observed differences also imply that further patterns will be uncovered as other orders are studied, and that, at present, general statements about mammalian embryogenesis can be only tentative at best.

General

Embryos were recovered from the genital tracts of spontaneously bred does at the indicated times *post coitum* by sacrificing the doe and flushing the genital tract with warm culture medium. Embryos exactly three days *post coitum* were present both in the distal oviduct and uterus, whereas earlier stages were entirely oviductal and later ones entirely uterine. To obtain sufficient material for reliable measurements on cleavage stage embryos, six month old virgin Dutch does were superovulated. Three weeks following a single intramuscular injection of 25 i.u. of Follutein (Squibb), the does were given 0.3 mg of F.S.H.-P (Armour) subcutaneously twice daily for three days. Spontaneous breeding almost invariably succeeded the following day, and 2.5 mg P.L.H. (Calbiochem) was given into an ear vein immediately after breeding. An average of 28 embryos was recovered from each superovulated doe.

The embryos were exposed to radioisotope in F-10 medium (Ham, '63) contained in open watch glasses and maintained at 37.5–38.0° in an atmosphere of 5% carbon dioxide in air at saturation humidity. In contrast to its reported enhancing effect on radioisotope uptake in mouse embryos (Woodland and Graham, '69) and on protein synthesis in rabbit blastocysts (Manes and Daniel. '69), serum protein had no consistently demonstrable effect on uridine or thymidine uptake in preimplantation rabbit embryos and was omitted from the medium for better definition of the experimental conditions.

Embryos were exposed either to thymidine-methyl-H^3 (19.2 c/mM) or to uridine-H^3 (10.3 c/mM) at a concentration of 20 μCi per ml for a standard two hour period. In the experiments in which inhibitors of nucleic acid synthesis were employed, the embryos were exposed to Actinomycin D simultaneously with the radioisotope, whereas a 30 minute pre-exposure to Mitomycin C was allowed, since this compound must be metabolized to its reduced form for optimal inhibitory activity (Iyer and Szybalski, '63; Lipsett and Weissbach, '65).

Ham's F-10 medium without phenol red was obtained from Hyland Laboratories. Radioisotope-labeled compounds were obtained from New England Nuclear Corporation. Actinomycin D was obtained as "Lyovac Cosmegen" from Merck, Sharp, and Dohme; Mitomycin C was obtained from Sigma Chemical Company.

Preparation of embryos for liquid scintillation counting

Following exposure to the radioisotope, the embryos were prepared for liquid scintillation counting essentially as described previously (Manes and Daniel, '69). Briefly, the method involves washing the embryos in chilled, non-radioactive medium three times, then lysing them in sodium dodecyl sulfate-urea, precipitating the acid-insoluble materials with trichloroacetic acid, then collecting and washing this precipitate on filters, which are dried and counted under a toluene-PPO-POPOP scintillation mixture. Two alterations were made in the procedure for the present study: (1) the enzyme Pronase (B grade, Calbiochem) was used to digest the embryos, and only in the presence of SDS-urea, so that contaminating nucleases were inactivated; and (2) the hot trichloroacetic acid extraction was omitted.

Counting was carried out in Picker Liquimat at a tritium efficiency of approximately 42%.

Determination of orcinol-reactive materials in embryos

Embryos for these determinations were flushed from the genital tract with isotonic saline, counted, washed briefly in distilled water, and transferred in a small volume to a 1.0 ml centrifuge tube treated with Desicote (Beckman). Large blastocysts were washed in saline, drained and placed in the centrifuge tubes singly, where they were ruptured with a stainless steel wire and centrifuged at 3000 g for ten minutes, and the supernatant blastocoelic fluid was then removed. The embryos were stored at −20° until samples of all preimplantation stages had been collected. They were then lyophilized and dissolved in 100 μl of 0.01 M EDTA, 1% sodium dodecyl sulfate pH7.0. Ten microliters of 5M sodium chloride and 200 μl of cold 95% ethanol were added and the mixture was allowed to stand overnight at −20°. The tubes were then centrifuged at 10,000 g for ten minutes, the supernatant carefully removed with a micropipette and the residue taken up in 40 μl of the EDTA-SDS buffer.

A micromodification of the orcinol reaction as described by Morse and Carter ('49) was employed. To the embryo sample, 100 μl of 0.02% ferric chloride in 10N hydrochloric acid and 10 μl of 6% orcinol in 95% ethanol were added. The tubes were heated in a boiling water bath for 20 minutes, cooled, centrifuged at 10,000 g for ten minutes and the optical density of the supernatant determined at 660 mμ using Beckman Microcells in a Gilford Model 2000 Spectrophotometer fitted with a Beckman Model DU light source. The "blank" optical density in this system was 0.032. A standard curve was prepared using purified HeLa cell RNA, and assuming an optical density of 1.00 at 260 mμ to represent 40 μg RNA/ml. The O.D.$_{260}$/O.D.$_{280}$ ratio of this RNA preparation was 2.09.

RESULTS

Incorporation of thymidine-methyl-H³ and uridine-H³ by preimplantation rabbit embryos

The measurements of radioactivity in acid-insoluble material obtained from embryos exposed to these two compounds for two hours in vitro are tabulated in table 1. Embryos were taken from the doe within 30 minutes of the times indicated post coitum. Thymidine-methyl-H³ incorporation was found to be insensitive to Actinomycin D at the concentration used but was found to be variably sensitive to Mitomycin C under the conditions described. It appeared to be as sensitive to Mitomycin C at a concentration of 10 μg per ml as at 100 μg per ml although the latter concentration has been reported necessary for the maximal effect in animal cells (Iyer and Szybalski, '63).

Uridine-H³ incorporation was more uniformly sensitive to Actinomycin D inhibition, the suppression falling generally between 89–95%, although the values at two days (80%) and six days (82%) are lower. The 2 μg per ml concentration was used since previous investigation has shown this to be the lowest concentration

TABLE 1

Incorporation of Uridine-H³ and Thymidine-methyl-H³ into acid-insoluble material by preimplantation rabbit embryos in vitro

Age of embryo at time of exposure to radioisotope (in days post coitum)	Number of cells per embryo [1]	Uridine-H³ incorporation CPM/embryo [2]		Thymidine-methyl-H³ incorporation CPM/embryo
		No actinomycin D	Actinomycin D, 2 μg/ml	Actinomycin D, 2 μg/ml
Unfertilized ova	1	0.20 ± 0.07 (27,25) [3]	0.17 (25)	0.16 (116)
1	2	10.6 ± 0.8 (28,40)	0.61 ± 0.06 (15,40,20)	1.5 (146)
2	16	26.3 ± 2.6 (25,17,35,39,47,65)	5.3 ± 2.18 (20,32)	27 (140)
3	128	1,258 ± 106 (18,16,3,30,10,6,9)	71 ± 26 (19,5,10)	359 ± 12 (14,10)
4	1,024	9,720 ± 190 (24,7)	1,158 ± 186 (25,7)	1,884 ± 168 (6,10)
5	9,000	12,540 ± 894 (12,9,7)	1,133 ± 33 (10,7)	12,520 (7)
6	80,000	24,750 ± 4760 (4,4,4,4,3,2)	4,475 ± 688 (4,4,4,2)	15,580 ± 1590 (4,4,3,3)

[1] See Daniel, '64.
[2] Expressed as weighted means ± standard error.
[3] Numbers in parentheses are the number of embryos pooled for each determination.

capable of producing maximum suppression of uridine-H³ incorporation in the six day blastocyst (Manes, unpublished data).

The Actinomycin D-insensitive incorporation of uridine -H³ is presumed to be incorporation into DNA and into the terminal -CCA sequence of tRNA through metabolism to cytidine and thymidine, since the uridine used was generally labeled.

As the molecular weights of these two compounds are nearly identical (thymidine, 242.2; uridine, 244.2), and their chemistries closely related, it would be expected that variations in embryonic permeabilities during the preimplantation period should affect the uptake of these compounds equally. It can be seen in table 1 that the rates of incorporation of the two compounds do not follow the same pattern during this period, and the most likely explanation for this phenomenon is the different uses to which they are put by the embryo. The methyl labeling of thymidine, and the sensitivity of its incorporation to inhibition by Mitomycin C but not by Actinomycin D are consistent with its incorporation exclusively into DNA. The Actinomycin D-sensitive incorporation of uridine-H³ is, by all evidence available, solely into RNA.

The incorporation data are presented in table 1 as counts per minute per embryo. Although cleavage during the first two days is reasonably synchronous, synchrony is lost by the third day and there is progressive variability in embryonic size and stage of development over the remaining days of the preimplantation period. The mean number of cells per embryo throughout this period has been determined (Daniel, '64) and one can reduce the effect of biological variability on the quantitation of DNA and RNA synthesis by presenting the incorporation data as counts per minute per embryonic cell. This information is presented graphically in figure 1. These counts are total thymidine incorporation less machine background and only Actinomycin D-sensitive uridine incorporation. The striking difference in the patterns of incorporation of these two compounds is evident, uridine incorporation showing two prominent peaks: immediately after fertilization and on the third day *post coitum*.

The significance of this pattern will be discussed below.

The presentation of data in figure 1 suffers from the fact that, following blastocyst formation, the embryo consists of at least two different kinds of cells, those of the trophoblast and those of the inner cell mass. The synthetic activities of these two cell types were not evaluated separately in the present study and future investigation may show them to be quite different.

Content of orcinol-reactive material in preimplantation rabbit embryos

Measurements of synthetic processes in mammalian embryos *in vitro* have been subjected to the criticism that these data may not reflect the true *in vivo* state of affairs, and that *in vitro* conditions may alter embryonic permeabilities or affect the incorporation of exogenous materials in some other way. For this reason, it is desirable to have some measure of synthetic processes that is independent of the

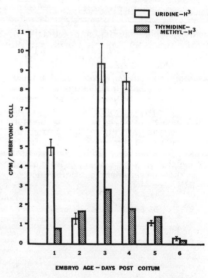

Fig. 1 Pattern of incorporation of uridine-H³ and thymidine-methyl-H³ by preimplantation rabbit embryos *in vitro*. Standard errors are shown only for uridine-H³ incorporation, since multiple determinations of thymidine-methyl-H³ were not generally carried out.

183

in vitro incorporation data. The determinations of orcinol-reactive material in the embryos fulfill this requirement and these data are given in table 2. The orcinol reaction appears to be quite specific for ribose, although interference with the reaction by other biological materials has been reported (Hutchison and Munro, '61). Calf thymus DNA did not contribute detectably to the color formation in the present method, and the ethanol precipitation was used to remove soluble ribose-containing material from the reaction mixture. Thus, the values given here should closely estimate the RNA polymer content of rabbit embryos during the preimplantation period. It is of interest to note that the six day mean value of 2.79 µg per embryo can be calculated to represent 35×10^{-12} gm RNA per embryonic cell, given an embryo of 80,000 cells (Daniel, '64). This value compares favorably with the $25–30 \times 10^{-12}$ gm RNA per HeLa cell obtained by McConkey and Hopkins ('64).

DISCUSSION

The incorporation of uridine-H^3 into acid-insoluble material, and estimates of emybryonic RNA content, provide clues to the metabolism of RNA in preimplantation rabbit embryos. It is evident, for example, that there is no detectable incorporation of labeled uridine into unfertilized ova, whereas within 12 hours after fertilization (24 hours following coitus) significant incorporation is occurring. In spite of measurable incorporation during the cleavage period, however, there is no increase in embryonic RNA content until 72 hours *post coitum*. It is precisely at this time that acceleration of uridine incorpo-

ration is demonstrated, and that the transformation of the morula into a blastocyst begins as the embryo leaves the oviduct and enters the uterus.

The data indicate that cleavage of the rabbit ovum results in a progressive decrease in the RNA content of each successive blastomere. The unfertilized ovum contains approximately 20 nanograms of RNA, whereas each blastomere at the 16-cell stage contains but 2.1 nanograms. A similar phenomenon has been reported in cleaving mouse embryos (Reamer, '63) and in cleaving rat embryos (Austin and Braden, '53). Not surprisingly, the large rabbit ovum appears to contain approximately ten times as much RNA as the mouse ovum.

From these combined observations, it may be tentatively concluded that cleavage of the mammalian egg can be accomplished without net RNA synthesis. These observations suggest further that stable RNA species, ribosomal and transfer RNAs, are not synthesized during early cleavage, and, indeed, these syntheses are not detectable in mouse embryos before the 4-cell stage (Woodland and Graham, '69). The mature mammalian oocyte, in spite of its diminutive size, is thus probably equipped with sufficient stores of these forms of RNA to carry the embryo through at least the initial stages of cleavage, in a manner somewhat comparable to that demonstrated in non-mammalian embryogenesis (Gross, '67). When these syntheses become absolutely *necessary* for continued mammalian development, as opposed to when they actually occur, is still an open question.

TABLE 2

Ribonucleic acid content of rabbit embryos during the preimplantation period

Age of embryo (in days *post coitum*)	Number of embryos pooled for each determination	RNA content per embryo, in micrograms (weighted mean ± standard error)
Unfertilized ova	50, 43, 45, 45, 65	0.020 ± 0.002
1	50, 57, 75	0.028 ± 0.003
2	36, 58, 61	0.034 ± 0.002
3	20, 19, 21, 25, 25	0.069 ± 0.005
4	15, 18, 16	0.123 ± 0.008
5	5, 5, 6, 10	0.414 ± 0.027
6	1, 1, 1, 1, 1, 1, 1	2.79 ± 0.20

The extreme sensitivity of the mouse egg to Actinomycin D (Mintz, '64; Thomson and Biggers, '66) argues in favor of at least some necessary RNA synthesis immediately following fertilization. Cleavage of the 2-cell mouse egg is inhibited by the antibiotic at 10^{-7}M concentrations. Rabbit ova, which can be cultured from the single cell stage, are inhibited from cleaving by this same concentration (Manes, unpublished data). This concentration is far below that used for maximum suppression of uridine incorporation in the present experiments, and has been shown to suppress ribosomal and transfer RNA synthesis in the preimplantation mouse embryo without significantly affecting the synthesis of DNA-like RNA (Ellem and Gwatkin, '68). It should be pointed out, however, that Actinomycin D inhibits cleavage *before* the synthesis of either ribosomal or transfer RNA can be detected in the mouse embryo. There would thus appear to be two possible explanations for the inhibitory action of the antibiotic: either (1) there is some synthesis of non-ribosomal and non-transfer RNA immediately following fertilization which is extremely sensitive to the antibiotic and which is necessary for cleavage or (2) the antibiotic may be interfering with cleavage by some means other than its well-known interference with DNA-dependent RNA synthesis.

Evidence which opposes the first explanation stems from an alternative method of interfering with nucleic acid metabolism in cleaving mammalian embryos. Adams, Hay and Lutwak-Mann ('61) found that purine analogues administered to the pregnant rabbit during the time of ovum fertilization and early embryonic development had no effect on the normal progression of cleavage. They found however that even brief exposure of the embryo to these substances during cleavage resulted in abnormalities in blastocyst development several days later. They have, in sum, demonstrated that the effect of these purine analogues is not immediate but delayed. Since the present data show that Actinomycin D-sensitive incorporation of uridine is occurring is cleaving rabbit embryos, the evidence to date is consistent with the notion that this RNA synthesis is not required for cleavage but is in preparation for later differentiative events, again comparable to what is known of non-mammalian embryogenesis (Brown and Littna '66; Infante and Nemer, '67). The deleterious effects of Actinomycin D on cleavage of the mammalian egg may therefore quite conceivably be due to other actions of the drug (Honig and Rabinovitz, '65; Laszlo et al., '66).

The acceleration of uridine-H^3 incorporation by the preimplantation rabbit embryo at 72 hours *post coitum* shown above precedes the acceleration of amino acids-C^{14} incorporation by some 36 hours (Manes and Daniel, '69). This relationship differs considerably from that found in the preimplantation mouse embryo (Monesi and Salfi, '67), in which the incorporation of both leucine and lysine increased some 12–24 hours before an increase in uridine incorporation was detected. Other data on synthetic events in the preimplantation mouse (Mintz, '64; Woodland and Graham, '69) demonstrate, however, an acceleration in RNA synthesis at the 4-cell stage, considerably earlier than that shown by Monesi and Salfi.

As has been pointed out previously (Manes and Daniel, '69), the acceleration of amino acid incorporation in the preimplantation rabbit embryo correlates well in time with other properties which appear in the embryo. Oxygen uptake increases markedly on the fourth day *post coitum* (Fridhandler, '61), the embryo is capable of utilizing glucose as sole carbon source for the first time (Daniel, '67), and sex chromatin becomes detectable (Melander, '62). It is of interest, also, that rabbit embryos artificially retained in the oviduct or developing in ovariectomized mothers (Adams, '58; Adams, '65), or cultured in serum-depleted media (Pincus and Werthessen, '38), appear to arrest at the mid-blastocyst stage of development, that stage at which the acceleration of protein synthesis would normally occur. Although the phenomenon of "embryonic diapause" has not been seen in the rabbit, the reversible arrest of embryonic development at the mid-blastocyst stage in many mammals is difficult to interpret without invoking environmental "factors" capable of regulating embryonic events.

These observations suggest that the embryo places rather stringent requirements upon the environment in order to accomplish this acceleration in protein synthesis, and further that this protein synthesis is a *sine qua non* for further development and differentiation. What these requirements are is, at the moment, a matter for speculation. By way of contrast, preliminary data in this laboratory indicate that the acceleration of uridine incorporation at 72 hours *post coitum* is not prevented by ovariectomy or by retention in the oviduct.

For these reasons, a tentative working model of molecular embryogenesis during the preimplantation period in the mammal is hereby proposed. The model is heavily indebted to evidence derived from other sources (Spirin, '66; Tyler, '67) which indicates the fairly general phenomenon of "stored" informational RNA, and the phenomenon of "post-transcriptional" regulation of protein synthesis in differentiating systems (Scherrer and Marcaud, '68). It is proposed that cleavage in the mammal is accomplished using "stored" maternal RNAs, and that early RNA synthesis in the embryo is in preparation for later differentiative events. It is further proposed that the initial transcription of the embryonic genome is not as critically dependent upon environmental "factors" as is translation of the message into the first embryonic proteins, and that this latter event is subject to "post-transcriptional" regulation by the maternal environment.

This model fits most of the known facts concerning preimplantation mammalian development. The broad outlines of the model, it is hoped, will at least provide a framework for meaningful experimentation.

ACKNOWLEDGMENTS

The technical assistance of Mrs. Mary White in completing the orcinol determinations is gratefully acknowledged. This work was supported by grant No. HD-04024-01 from the National Institutes of Health.

LITERATURE CITED

Adams, C. E. 1958 Egg development in the rabbit: the influence of post-coital ligation of the uterine tube and of ovariectomy. J. Endocrin., 16: 283–293.

——— 1965 The influence of maternal environment on preimplantation stages of pregnancy in the rabbit. In: Preimplantation Stages of Pregnancy. G. W. Wolstenholme and M. O'Connor, eds. Little, Brown, and Co., Boston, pp. 345–373.

Adams, C. E., M. F. Hay and C. Lutwak-Mann 1961 The action of various agents upon the rabbit embryo. J. Embryol. Exp. Morph., 9: 468–491.

Austin, C. R., and A. W. H. Braden 1953 The distribution of nucleic acids in rat eggs in fertilization and early segmentation. Aust. J. Biol. Sci., 6: 324–334.

Brown, D. D., and E. Littna 1966 Synthesis and accumulation of DNA-like RNA during embryogenesis of Xenopus laevis. J. Mol. Biol., 20: 81–94.

Daniel, J. C., Jr. 1964 Early growth of rabbit trophoblast. Amer. Natur., 98: 85–87.

——— 1967 The pattern of utilization of respiratory metabolic intermediates by preimplantation rabbit embryos in vitro. Exp. Cell Res., 47: 619–624.

Ellem, K. A. O., and R. B. L. Gwatkin 1968 Patterns of nucleic acid synthesis in the early mouse embryo. Develop. Biol., 18: 311–330.

Fridhandler, L. 1961 Pathways of glucose metabolism in fertilized rabbit ova at various preimplantation stages. Exp. Cell Res., 22: 303–316.

Gross, P. R. 1967 RNA metabolism in embryonic development and differentiation. New England J. Med., 276: 1239–1247, 1297–1305.

Ham, R. G. 1963 An improved nutrient solution for diploid Chinese hamster and human cell lines. Exp. Cell Res., 29: 515–526.

Honig, G. R., and M. Rabinovitz 1965 Actinomycin-D inhibition of protein synthesis unrelated to effect on template RNA synthesis. Science, 149: 1504–1506.

Hutchison, W. C., and H. N. Munro 1961 The determination of nucleic acids in biological materials. Analyst, 86: 768–813.

Infante, A. A., and M. Nemer 1967 Accumulation of newly synthesized RNA templates in a unique class of polyribosomes during embryogenesis. Proc. Natl. Acad. Sci. U. S., 58: 681–688.

Iyer, V. N., and W. Szybalski 1963 A molecular mechanism of Mitomycin action: linking of complementary DNA strands. Proc. Natl. Acad. Sci. U. S., 50: 355–362.

Laszlo, J., D. S. Miller, K. S. McCarty and P. Hochstein 1966 Actinomycin D: inhibition of respiration and glycolysis. Science, 151: 1007–1010.

Lipsett, M. N., and A. Weissbach 1965 The site of alkylation of nucleic acids by Mitomycin. Biochem., 4: 206–211.

Manes, C., and J. C. Daniel, Jr. 1969 Quantitative aspects of protein synthesis in the preimplantation rabbit embryo. Exptl. Cell Res., 55: 261–268.

McConkey, E. H., and J. W. Hopkins 1964 The relationship of the nucleolus to the synthesis of ribosomal RNA in HeLa cells. Proc. Natl. Acad. Sci. U. S., 51: 1197–1204.

Melander, Y. 1962 Chromosomal behavior during the origin of sex chromatin in the rabbit. Hereditas, 48: 645–661.

Mintz, B. 1964 Synthetic processes and early development in the mammalian egg. J. Exp. Zool., 157: 85–100.

Monesi, V., and V. Salfi 1967 Macromolecular syntheses during early development in the mouse embryo. Exp. Cell Res., 46: 632–635.

Morse, M. L., and C. E. Carter 1949 The synthesis of nucleic acids in cultures of *Escherichia coli*, strains B and B/R. J. Bacteriology, 58: 317–326.

Pincus, G., and N. T. Werthessen 1938 The comparative behavior of mammalian eggs *in vivo* and *in vitro*. J. Exp. Zool., 78: 1–18.

Reamer, G. R. 1963 The quantity and distribution of nucleic acids in the early cleavage stages of the mouse embryo. Ph.D. Thesis, Boston University, 108 pp.

Scherrer, K., and L. Marcaud 1968 Messenger RNA in avian erythroblasts at the transcriptional and translational levels and the problem of regulation in animal cells. J. Cell Physiol., 72 (Suppl. 1): 181–212.

Spirin, A. S. 1966 On "masked" forms of messenger RNA in early embryogenesis and in other differentiating systems. In: Current Topics in Developmental Biology. A. Monroy and A. A. Moscona, eds. Academic Press, New York, pp. 2–38.

Thomson, J. L., and J. D. Biggers 1966 Effect of inhibitors of protein synthesis on the development of preimplantation mouse embryos. Exp. Cell Res., 41: 411–427.

Tyler, A. 1967 Masked messenger RNA and cytoplasmic DNA in relation to protein synthesis and processes of fertilization and determination in embryonic development. Develop. Biol., 16 (Suppl. 1): 170–226.

Woodland, H. R., and C. F. Graham 1969 RNA synthesis during early development of the mouse. Nature, 221: 327–332.

Nucleic Acid Synthesis in Preimplantation Rabbit Embryos

II. DELAYED SYNTHESIS OF RIBOSOMAL RNA

COLE MANES

The mammalian zygote undergoes a period of cleavage, during which the maternally-inherited cytoplasm is parceled into progressively smaller units, before true growth begins with the transformation of the morula into a blastocyst. The extent to which the embryonic genome is utilized during this early period is not known, but it might be predicted that the requirements for genetic expression during cleavage would be considerably less than the requirements during a period of logarithmic growth in which cell differentiation becomes evident. It has been previously shown (Manes, '69) that synthesis of ribonucleic acid (RNA) in rabbit embryos accelerates markedly at the beginning of the growth period, and that there is also a rapid increase in total embryonic RNA content at this time. The present studies were undertaken for the purpose of characterizing the species of RNA involved in this transition in early rabbit development, as potential indicators of changing utilization of the embryonic genome.

During the past few years, a number of investigators have taken advantage of the capability of polyacrylamide gels in the electrophoretic separation of RNA species by molecular sieving (Grossbach and Weinstein, '68; Loening, '67; Bishop et al., '67; Peacock and Dignman, '67). The present studies are also based upon this technique, which provides a simple, rapid, and accurate method for analyzing the synthetic patterns in limited amounts of biological material. Combined with the technique of radioisotope labeling of embryonic RNA *in vitro*, under conditions which allow apparently normal growth during the short labeling period, the method has provided a means of examing the synthesis of stable, homogeneous RNA species in rabbit embryos during the preimplantation period.

Previous studies of the RNA synthesized by the preimplantation mammal have utilized the mouse embryo and the techniques of MAK column chromatography and sucrose density gradient sedimentation (Ellem and Gwatkin, '68; Woodland

and Graham, '69; Piko, '70; Monesi et al., '70). The synthesis of both ribosomal and transfer RNA (rRNA and tRNA) is detectable at the 4-cell stage of cleavage in the mouse embryo by these methods, as was suggested by the autoradiographic findings of Mintz ('64). The very early synthesis of these two gene products, together with the inhibitory effects of low concentrations of Actinomycin D on cleavage of the mouse egg (Mintz, '64; Thomson and Biggers, '66), has prompted the conclusion that mammalian embryogenesis requires essentially immediate genetic intervention, in contrast with most non-mammalian systems (Gross, '67).

The results of the investigations of RNA metabolism in the preimplantation rabbit embryo to be presented here suggest that the small mouse embryo may not be the typical mammalian system. The rabbit egg cleaves to a morula of 100-130 cells before initiating rRNA synthesis at the beginning of the growth period, whereas the synthesis of tRNA is detectable from the onset of cleavage. The clear separation of these two syntheses in time is consistent with their independent regulation in the rabbit embryo, and is reminiscent of the constant tRNA/DNA ratio found in bacterial systems (Kjeldgaard and Kurland, '63), where the rRNA/DNA ratio is proportional to growth rate.

MATERIALS AND METHODS

General

Embryos were collected from superovulated Dutch rabbits or from normally-bred New Zealand or California rabbits by methods previously described (Manes, '69). The embryos were immediately placed in 0.5-2.0 ml of F-10 medium (Ham, '63) containing uridine-5-H[3] (New England Nuclear Corp.) at a concentration of 200 microcuries per milliliter. Incorporation of the radioisotope was generally allowed for four to six hours, as indicated. In those experiments involving Actinomycin D ("Lyovac Cosmegen," Merck, Sharp and Dohme), embryos were exposed to the antibiotic and to the radioisotope simultaneously. The embryos were then washed twice in cold isotonic saline and stored at $-20°$ for no longer than 72 hours before use. Ten milligrams

frozen rabbit liver was added as carrier during the nucleic acid extraction.

Extraction of RNA

The embryos and carrier liver tissue were homogenized at 0-4° in the sucrose-Tris buffer pH 7.4 described by Loening ('65). The homogenate was centrifuged at 20,000 g for 15 minutes to remove whole cells, nuclei, mitochondria, and lysosomes. The supernatant was made 0.01 M EDTA, triisopropyl naphthalene sulfonic acid (TNS, sodium salt, Eastman Organic) was added to a final concentration of 5%, and the mixture brought to room temperature and stirred for 15-20 minutes.

Nucleic acids were extracted at 55° using the phenol-cresol mixture described by Kirby ('65). After 15 minutes, an equal volume of chloroform containing 1% isoamyl alcohol was added (Penman, '66), the mixture again brought briefly to 55°, and then centrifuged at room temperature at 700 g for two minutes. The lower phase was removed, and the aqueous phase re-extracted as above. Again the lower phase was removed, 1/10 volume of 30% sodium chloride was added to the aqueous phase, and the extraction repeated. The aqueous phase was finally extracted three times with the chloroform-isoamyl alcohol mixture alone, then nucleic acids were precipitated from the aqueous phase by the addition of 2.5 volumes of 95% ethanol at $-20°$. Precipitation was allowed for two hours or overnight at $-20°$, and the nucleic acid precipitate was collected by centrifugation at 10,000 g for ten minutes.

The TNS detergent was co-precipitated with the nucleic acids by this method, and its removal was found to be essential for optimal separation and staining of the RNA in the polyacrylamide gels. The method described by Kirby ('65) for the selective precipitation of polysaccarides from solutions of nucleic acids using tetraethyl ammonium bromide proved quite effective for removing the TNS, the RNA being precipitated under these conditions and the TNS remaining in the supernatant. Precipitation in 50% ethanol alone was also effective, but the sample did not yield the clean electrophoretic separations

189

obtained by the tetraethyl ammonium bromide procedure. The almost invisible precipitate was again pelleted by centrifugation and dried in a vacuum.

Electrophoresis of RNA

The electrophoresis system was essentially that described by Loening ('67). The RNA sample was taken up in electrode buffer containing 10% sucrose to yield a solution of approximately 1 microgram RNA per microliter. The entire sample dissolved in 40 μliters, and was heated to 70° for four minutes immediately before electrophoresis. The sample was divided equally between two cylindrical 2.5% polyacrylamide gels measuring 4 × 55 mm, which had been pre-run in electrode buffer for 60 minutes. Electrophoresis was carried out at room temperature, 2.5 ma per gel, for 60 minutes. At the end of the run, the gels were placed in cold 6% acetic acid for ten minutes, then stained for one hour in 0.2% methylene blue in a sodium acetate-acetic acid buffer (Peacock and Dingman, '68).

After de-staining in deionized water, the gels were scanned in a modified Photovolt Model 52C Densitometer fitted with a 610 millimicron wavelength filter.

Radioactivity measurement in gel fractions

Gels were frozen and sliced into 1.5 mm fractions. Each fraction was placed in a separate scintillation vial (Beckman) and allowed to dry over-night. The gel fractions were then processed for liquid scintillation counting by the method of Tishler and Epstein ('68), using a toluene-PPO-POPOP cocktail (5.0 gm 2,5-diphenyloxazole, 0.1 gm p-bis-2 (5-phenyloxazolyl) benzene in toluene to 1 l). Counting was carried out in a Beckman Model LS-100 scintillation counter at a tritium efficiency of 40%.

Preparation of marker RNA

Rabbit liver was homogenized in the sucrose-Tris buffer described above, and centrifuged at 20,000 g for 15 minutes. The supernatant was then subjected to centrifugation at 105,000 g for 60 min-

utes in a Spinco Model L centrifuge. Nucleic acids were extracted separately from the supernatant and from the ribosomal pellet, and electrophoresis carried out as described above.

28S HeLa cell RNA, prepared by cold phenol extraction and sucrose density gradient centrifugation, was kindly supplied by Dr. E. H. McConkey.

RESULTS

Identification of cytoplasmic RNA species

RNA molecules up to 30S in size will enter polyacrylamide gels of 2.5% total acrylamide concentration under the electrophoretic conditions employed (Loening, '67). Figure 1a illustrates the three major bands obtained when total cytoplasmic RNA is separated under the conditions described above. Figure 1b demonstrates that the band 53-55 mm from the origin is essentially the only RNA found in the high speed supernatant (S), whereas the two prominent bands at 9-10 mm and at 21-22 mm are associated only with the ribosomal pellet (RP). Figure 1c, showing only a single band, illustrates the migration of HeLa cell 28S RNA under these conditions, and identifies the band at 9-10 mm as the RNA from the heavier ribosomal subunit.

The RNA from the smaller ribosomal subunit, found at 21-22 mm, will by convention be referred to as 18S, and that at 53-55 mm as 4S or transfer RNA (tRNA). These migratory properties are in good general agreement with those published previously (Loening, '67; Bishop et al., '67).

Multiple minor bands were visible in the original gels, but do not show in the photographs. The 5S ribosomal RNA component is visible, however, at 49-51 mm in the ribosomal pellet (RP) sample.

When nucleic acid preparations were carried out to include nuclear and mitochondrial DNA, by omitting the initial centrifugation at 20,000 g, a sharp band with a violet color was found at 4-5 mm from the origin. This band was eliminated by prior treatment of the sample with purified DNAse (Worthington, RNAse-free), whereas none of the other bands was affected by DNAse treatment.

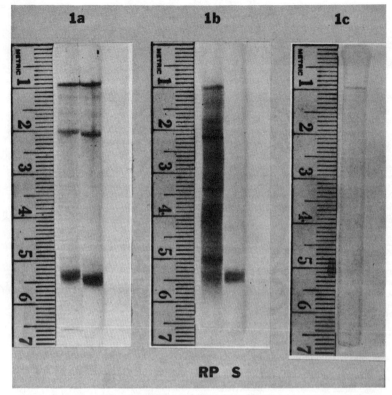

Fig. 1 Separation of cytoplasmic RNA in 2.5% polyacrylamide gels. (a) Total cytoplasmic RNA. (b) RNA extracted from 105,000 g pellet (RP) and supernatant (S). (c) HeLa cell 28S RNA.

Incorporation of uridine-5-H³ into cytoplasmic RNA species by preimplantation rabbit embryos

The patterns of incorporation in rabbit embryos during the first six days of development, when labeled *in vitro* under the conditions indicated, are shown in figures 2 through 7. All experiments were repeated at least once with essentially identical results. There is some shift in the positions of the major peaks from one gel to another, due primarily to current fluctuations during the earlier electrophoretic runs. The significant considera-

tion, however, is the correspondence of incorporation peaks with the major optical density peaks. Furthermore, only the qualitative aspect of these patterns is to be emphasized, and no quantitative information as to relative rates of incorporation into various species can be inferred. There is, as yet, no information as to the relative specific activities of the nucleoside triphosphate pools in these embryos. The period of exposure to the radiosotope exaggerates the resulting total incorporation into stable RNA. Likewise, labeling with uridine-5-H³, while preventing the labeling of DNA, produces greater incor-

191

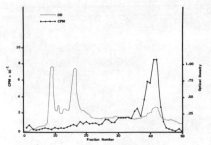

Fig. 2 Pattern of uridine-5-H³ incorporation by rabbit embryos labeled 24-29 hours *post coitum* (140 embryos).

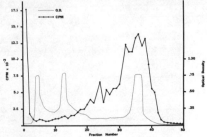

Fig. 4 Pattern of uridine-5-H³ incorporation by rabbit embryos labeled 67-72 hours *post coitum* (87 embryos).

poration of the radioisotope into those RNA species having relatively high uridine content. Thus, rRNA, with approximately 20% uridine, would tend to be more heavily labeled than tRNA, having approximately 15% uridine (Gross et al., '65).

The most striking feature of these patterns is the absence of detectable incorporation into 28S and 18S peaks prior to 72 hours *post coitum*. Even those embryos exposed to the radioisotope between 67 and 72 hours *post coitum* (fig. 4), which is within the eight hour period required for cell division at this stage (Daniel, '64), show no incorporation into cytoplasmic rRNA peaks. This pattern of incorporation just prior to 72 hours *post coitum*, however, as well as that immediately following (fig. 5), does reveal some incorporation into high molecular weight RNA which is retained at the origin of the gels. Al-

though the extraction procedure followed in these experiments tends to minimize nuclear contamination, the freezing and thawing of the embryos may well allow some "leakage" of nuclear RNA, which would presumably account for RNA of this size. It is probable that at least some of this high molecular weight RNA is rRNA precursor (Piko, '70). The characterization of nuclear RNA synthesis in these embryos will be the subject of a later communication.

In contrast to the absence of rRNA synthesis prior to 72 hours *post coitum*, there is detectable incorporation of radioisotope into the 4S peak by the 2-cell embryo at 24 hours *post coitum*. The total incorporation in the 2-cell embryo is quite low, but by 48 and 72 hours *post coitum* incorporation into the 4S region is prominent. The overall pattern of incorporation established in the 72 hour

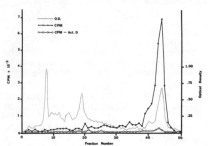

Fig. 3 Pattern of uridine-5-H³ incorporation by rabbit embryos labeled 48-54 hours *post coitum* (53 embryos, control; 100 embryos in Actinomycin D, 2 μg/ml).

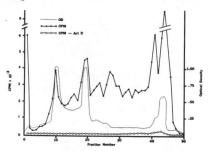

Fig. 5 Pattern of uridine-5-H³ incorporation by rabbit embryos labeled 72-77 hours *post coitum* (30 embryos, control; 17 embryos in Actinomycin D, 2 μg/ml).

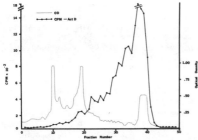

Fig. 6 Pattern of uridine-5-H³ incorporation by rabbit embryos labeled 74-79 hours *post coitum* in Actinomycin D 0.04 μg/ml (35 embryos).

embryo, which is the very beginning of blastocyst formation, persists throughout the remainder of the preimplantation period (fig. 7), although rates of incorporation continue to increase.

Whether the very early incorporation of radioisotope into 4S RNA represents unequivocal synthesis of functioning, mature tRNA is not clear from these experiments. However, incorporation into this peak at 48 and 72 hours is severely inhibited by Actinomycin D at 2 μg per milliliter (figs. 3, 5), consistent with DNA-dependent synthesis of this material at these stages. In addition, minor Actinomycin D-resistant incorporation remains under this peak at both times, being further consistent with terminal -CCA cytoplasmic labeling of tRNA through conversion of the labeled uridine precursor to cytidine.

Actinomycin D, at 0.04 μg per milliliter, was reported by Perry ('63) to in-

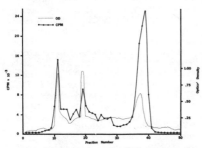

Fig. 7 Pattern of uridine-5-H³ incorporation by rabbit embryos labeled 144-147 hours *post coitum* (25 embryos).

hibit nucleolar labeling of HeLa cells while leaving general chromatin labeling unaffected. Figure 6 shows the effect of this low concentration of Actinomycin D on incorporation in the 3-day rabbit embryo. It is evident that the low level of antibiotic blocks the incorporation into ribosomal peaks much more completely than that into other fractions of the gel. This selective sensitivity to Actinomycin D is further evidence of true rRNA synthesis in the three day embryo.

Incorporation into heterogeneous RNA, migrating between the 18S and 4S peaks, is detectable at all preimplantation stages, but becomes particularly prominent in the patterns obtained between 67 and 77 hours *post coitum*. The size distribution of this material is consistent with that of cytoplasmic informational RNA in animal cells. Incorporation in this region is likewise completely blocked by Actinomycin D at 2 μg per milliliter (figs. 3, 5).

DISCUSSION

The synthesis of rRNA during the cleavage period at a level below the limits of detection in these experiments is not ruled out, but its contribution to the total incorporation pattern at the time of the morula-to-blastocyst transformation increases abruptly, apparently within a single cell division. Thus, the interval of development closely surrounding 72 hours *post coitum* is at least partially characterized by the derepression of that portion of the genome coding for rRNA. This interval coincides with the previously demonstrated acceleration in RNA synthesis and with the increase in embryonic RNA content (Manes, '69). It appears that the rabbit embryo is capable of carrying out its seven cleavage divisions in the absence of detectable ribosomal synthesis. Since protein synthesis is known to be occurring during cleavage (Manes and Daniel, '69), it is presumably accomplished on polysomes whose ribosomes are of maternal origin. Such a conclusion is made plausible by the finding of abundant ribosome clusters in the cytoplasm of rabbit ova (Zamboni and Mastroianni, '66).

Since there is no acceleration in protein synthesis in these embryos until approximately 108 hours *post coitum* (Manes and Daniel, '69), it may be pertinent to ask why new rRNA synthesis occurs some 36 hours earlier. In this regard, two points should be considered: (1) the synthesis of a gene product does not always indicate that it is *required* at that developmental stage. As a relevant example, rRNA synthesis normally begins at the gastrula stage in *Xenopus*, whereas the anucleolate mutant develops to the swimming tadpole stage in the complete absence of rRNA synthesis (Brown and Gurdon, '64; Gross, '67). And (2), the appearance of labeled precursor in cytoplasmic rRNA peaks does not of itself indicate that functioning new ribosomes are being formed (Perry, '67; Osawa, '68). Nothing is known about the synthesis of ribosomal proteins during preimplantation rabbit development, nor about the rapidity with which these new ribosomes are involved in polysomes. These are important questions which will have to be answered.

The earlier finding of a near-constant amount of total embryonic RNA during the cleavage period of rabbit development (Manes, '69) would seem to contradict the finding in these experiments that 4S RNA is synthesized as early as the 2-cell stage. This new synthesis could, of course, be closely counterbalanced by the simultaneous degradation of previously synthesized RNA, yielding little net change in total embryonic RNA. Rake and Graham ('64) report a rapidly turning over component in the 4S RNA of L cells. And, as discussed above, the quantitative contribution of this 4S RNA incorporation to total RNA metabolism during the labeling period cannot be derived from the present experiments. A minor contribution might well be missed within the limits of accuracy of the orcinol determinations.

The separation of 4S and 5S RNA is not ideal in gels of this low polyacrylamide concentration. At all stages of preimplantation development, however, labeling of the 5S region is evident, becoming more prominent relative to the 4S region at 67 hours *post coitum* (fig. 4). If the 5S ribosomal RNA component is being synthesized coordinately with the 28S and 18S components, as appears to be the usual situation (Brown and Littna, '66), then the increase in labeling of the 5S region at this time is probably due to the earliest beginnings of ribosomal assembly.

The lack of sensitivity of this labeling to low concentrations of Actinomycin D (fig. 6) is also consistent with the recent findings of Perry and Kelley ('68). The labeling in the 5S region during cleavage is conceivably due to the presence of a precursor to 4S RNA (Woodland and Graham, '69).

The finding of label in a heterogeneous class of RNA between the 4S and 18S markers is suggestive of the synthesis of informational RNA even in the very earliest stages of cleavage. It is possible that some of this material in the older embryos is the result of the degradation of high molecular weight RNA. However, prior to 72 hours *post coitum*, since no high molecular weight RNA is apparently being synthesized, degradation artifacts are a less likely explanation. The lack of hard facts regarding the hybridizing properties of this RNA and its involvement in polysomes precludes further speculation as to its role in embryogenesis.

Mention should be made of possible artifacts produced by the extremely high concentration of radioisotope to which the embryos were exposed. Although eventual harmful effects from irradiation would almost certainly be seen, these effects would not likely be significant during the labeling times used here. The same concentration (200 μCi/ml) was used by Woodland and Graham ('69) in labeling the RNA of mouse embryos. For reasons similar to theirs, it is felt that this level of radioactivity did not introduce serious deviations into the metabolic patterns of the embryos during the labeling period: 2-cell embryos cleaved at the normal rate, three day morulae began cavitation normally, and six day blastocysts remained well expanded during exposure to the radioisotope for periods up to six hours.

It therefore appears that the rabbit and mouse embryo share the property of very early synthesis of 4S RNA (presumptive tRNA), while differing in the time of onset of rRNA synthesis. The syntheses of these two RNA species are initiated within the same cell cycle in the mouse embryo (Woodland and Graham, '69), whereas they are separated by some six cell divisions in the rabbit. The rabbit embryo accordingly displays more clearly the separate controls over the expression of these genes, as do the embryos of the frog (Brown, '64) and sea urchin (Gross, '64). The later onset of rRNA synthesis in the rabbit also demonstrates the autonomy of its cleavage in at least this one respect. The coincidence of significant rRNA synthesis in the rabbit with the beginning of cavitation and with entry of the embryo into the uterus offers the opportunity for investigating possible maternal controls over embryonic events. The recent finding by Piko ('70), that mouse embryos cultured from the 2-cell stage display rRNA synthesis by the 8-cell stage *in vitro*, lends support to the idea that the initiation of rRNA synthesis in the embryo may be largely independent of environmental direction.

The discrepancy in the timing of rRNA synthesis between the mouse and rabbit may reflect a genuine difference in the requirements of these two embryos for genetic intervention, as a consequence, perhaps, of the much greater store of maternally-formed cytoplasm inherited by the rabbit embryo. Or the difference may be more apparent than real. As pointed out above, the onset of a given synthetic event may not correspond to its requirement in development. Until more is learned about the entry of these early gene products into polysomes, the immediacy of their use in directing development can only be guessed.

ACKNOWLEDGMENTS

The author is indebted to Mrs. Virginia Boschen and to Mrs. Margaret Benton for their technical assistance. This work was supported by grants HD-0424-01 and 1-R01-HD0274-01 from the National Institutes of Health.

LITERATURE CITED

Bishop, D. H. L., J. R. Claybrook and S. Spiegelman 1967 Electrophoretic separation of viral nucleic acids on polyacrylamide gels. J. Mol. Biol., 26: 373-387.

Brown, D. D. 1964 RNA synthesis during amphibian development. J. Exp. Zool., 157: 101-114.

Brown, D. D., and J. B. Gurdon 1964 Absence of ribosomal RNA synthesis in the anucleolate mutant of *Xenopus laevis*. Proc. Nat. Acad. Sci. U.S., 51: 139-146.

Brown, D. D., and E. Littna 1966 Synthesis and accumulation of low molecular weight RNA during embryogenesis of *Xenopus laevis*. J. Mol. Biol., 20: 95-112.

Daniel, J. C., Jr. 1964 Early growth of rabbit trophoblast. Amer. Natur., 98: 85-87.

Ellem, K. A. O., and R. B. L. Gwatkin 1968 Patterns of nucleic acid synthesis in the early mouse embryo. Develop. Biol., 18: 311-330.

Gross, P. R. 1964 The immediacy of genomic control during early development. J. Exp. Zool., 157: 21-38.

——— 1967 RNA metabolism in embryonic development and differentiation. New England J. Med., 276: 1239-1247, 1297-1305.

Gross, P. R., K. Kraemer and L. I. Malkin 1965 Base composition of RNA synthesized during cleavage of the sea urchin embryo. Biochem. Biophys. Res. Comm., 18: 569-575.

Grossbach, U., and I. B. Weinstein 1968 Separation of ribonucleic acids by polyacrylamide gel electrophoresis. Anal. Biochem., 22: 311-320.

Ham, R. G. 1963 An improved nutrient solution for diploid Chinese hamster and human cell lines, Exp. Cell Res., 29: 515-526.

Kirby, K. S. 1965 Isolation and characterization of ribosomal ribonucleic acid. Biochem. J., 96: 266-269.

Kjeldgaard, N. O., and C. G. Kurland 1963 The distribution of soluble and ribosomal RNA as a function of growth rate. J. Mol. Biol., 6: 341-348.

Loening, U. E. 1965 Synthesis of messenger ribonucleic acid in excised pea-seedling root segments. Biochem. J., 97: 125-133.

——— 1967 The fractionation of high molecular weight ribonucleic acid by polyacrylamide gel electrophoresis. Biochem. J., 102: 251-257.

Manes, C. 1969 Nucleic acid synthesis in preimplantation rabbit embryos. I. Quantitative aspects, relationship to early morphogenesis and protein synthesis. J. Exp. Zool., 172: 303-310.

Manes, C., and J. C. Daniel, Jr. 1969 Quantitative and qualitative aspects of protein synthesis in the preimplantation rabbit embryo. Exp. Cell Res., 55: 261-268.

Mintz, B. 1964 Synthetic processes and early development in the mammalian egg. J. Exp. Zool., 157: 85-100.

Monesi, V., M. Molinaro, E. Spalletta and G. Davoli 1970 Effect of metabolic inhibitors on macromolecular synthesis and early development in the mouse embryo. Exp. Cell Res., 59: 197-206.

Osawa, S. 1968 Ribosome formation and structure. Ann. Rev. Biochem., 37: 109-130.

Peacock, A. C., and C. W. Dingman 1967 Resolution of multiple ribonucleic acid species by polyacrylamide gel electrophoresis. Biochemistry, 6: 1818-1827.

Penman, S. 1966 RNA metabolism in the HeLa cell nucleus. J. Mol. Biol., 17: 117-130.

Perry, R. P. 1963 Selective effects of Actinomycin D on the intracellular distribution of RNA synthesis in tissue culture cells. Exp. Cell Res., 29: 400-406.

——— 1967 The nucleolus and the synthesis of ribosomes. Prog. Nucleic Acid Res. Mol. Biol., 6: 219-257.

Perry, R. P., and D. E. Kelley 1968 Persistent synthesis of 5S RNA when production of 28S and 18S ribosomal RNA is inhibited by low doses of Actinomycin D. J. Cell Physiol., 72: 235-246.

Piko, L. 1970 Synthesis of macromolecules in early mouse embryos cultured *in vitro:* RNA, DNA, and a polysaccharide component. Develop. Biol., 21: 257-279.

Rake, A. V., and A. F. Graham 1964 Kinetics of incorporation of uridine-C14 into L cell RNA. Biophys. J., 4: 267-284.

Thomson, J. L., and J. D. Biggers 1966 Effect of inhibitors of protein synthesis on the development of preimplantation mouse embryos. Exp. Cell Res., 41: 411-427.

Tishler, P. V., and C. J. Epstein 1968 A convenient method of preparing polyacrylamide gels for liquid scintillation spectrometry. Anal. Biochem., 22: 89-98.

Woodland, H. R., and C. F. Graham 1969 RNA synthesis during early development of the mouse. Nature, 221: 327-332.

Zamboni, L., and L. Mastroianni, Jr. 1966 Electron microscope studies on rabbit ova. II. The penetrated tubal ovum. J. Ultrastructure Res., 14: 95-117.

196

QUANTITATIVE AND QUALITATIVE ASPECTS OF PROTEIN SYNTHESIS IN THE PREIMPLANTATION RABBIT EMBRYO

C. MANES and J. C. DANIEL, JR

The preimplantation development of the rabbit embryo can be divided into two phases of approx. equal duration: a cleavage phase, characterized by no overall growth of the embryo and by low metabolic activity; and a blastocyst phase, characterized by rapid growth and greatly increased metabolic activity. This appearance of new properties in the embryo as the morula becomes a blastocyst is a common feature of all mammalian embryos studied to date, and has become the focal point of several lines of investigation made possible by improvements in the techniques of mammalian embryo culture, particularly of the rabbit [9, 11] and the mouse [4, 28]. It has been shown in these in vitro studies, for example, that the ability of both the rabbit and mouse embryo to utilize glucose as the sole energy source begins early in the blastocyst period [5, 12]. Further, oxygen consumption by the rabbit embryo rises sharply at this time [15], and the rate of incorporation of radioisotopes into RNA and protein in mouse embryos markedly increases [28, 30]. This developmental event, therefore, appears to be one of considerable importance in the early history of the mammalian embryo.

An intriguing property of preimplantation rabbit development is that the morula-to-blastocyst transition is largely under maternal control. The transition occurs at about the time of the passage of the embryo from the oviduct into the uterine cavity. Adams [1] has demonstrated that preventing the entry of the embryo into the uterus results in small and abortive blastocyst formation. He also showed that removal of hormonal support by ovariectomy during the cleavage period produced the same effect. The presence of "uterine factors" regulating blastocyst development has long been suspected, and Krishnan & Daniel [24] have recently isolated a glycoprotein from rabbit uterine secretions which is present only during the period of blastocyst development and which is capable of stimulating cavitation of rabbit morulae in vitro.

The investigator is therefore confronted, at least in the rabbit embryo, with a significant developmental event that is largely under environmental control. In contrast to the developmental events during embryogenesis in non-mammalian systems, where both the stimulus for the event and the response are enclosed within the embryo, the mammalian embryo appears to have retained chiefly the responses and to have consigned some of the stimuli to the maternal environment during this preimplantation period, very much in the fashion that it has consigned its nutritional stores [5, 6, 12, 14]. It is the purpose of this presentation to describe one of these responses in the rabbit embryo; the protein synthetic response. It has become increasingly evident [17] that changing protein populations underlie the phenotypic changes in cells resulting in developmental events and differentiation. It therefore seems appropriate to examine the morula-to-blastocyst transition with respect to embryonic protein populations, realizing that these populations are the end-product of both synthetic and degradative processes.

Through the introduction of radioactive precursors into embryonic macromolecules in vitro, the rates and the products of embryonic synthetic processes may be evaluated. In the investigations to be described, this technique, combined with liquid scintillation counting and polyacrylamide gel electrophoresis, has been employed to provide both quantitative and qualitative information regarding protein synthesis in the rabbit embryo throughout the preimplantation period. We shall present evidence that the morula-to-blastocyst transition in the rabbit is accompanied by a change in protein synthetic rate, and that certain species of embryonic protein are more affected by this rate change than are others. Since it has been proposed that the mammalian embryo constitutes the only known exception to the general phenomenon of delayed genetic intervention in development [18, 28], we shall discuss our evidence with respect to its bearing on "gene utilization" by the preimplantation rabbit embryo.

MATERIALS AND METHODS

Embryo culture

Rabbit embryos for these experiments were obtained at the required times post coitum by sacrificing the does and flushing the genital tracts with warm culture medium.

Culture was carried out in watch glasses containing 0.5 to 1.0 ml of Hams F-10 solution [21] supplemented with 5 mg/ml of lyophilized rabbit serum protein. The embryos were maintained at 37.5 to 38.0°C in an atmosphere of 5% carbon dioxide in air at saturation humidity.

Labeling of the embryonic protein in vitro was accomplished with the mixture of 15 amino acids, uniformly labeled, as supplied by New England Nuclear Corp., either as ^{14}C-amino acids at 5 μc/ml of culture medium, or as ^{3}H-amino acids at 50 μc/ml. The duration of exposure to the radioisotope was 4 h.

Preparation of embryos for scintillation counting

For the quantitative determination of radioisotope incorporation, the embryos were processed for liquid scintillation counting by a modification of the filter paper technique of Mans & Novelli [27]. At the end of the 4 h exposure to radioisotope, the embryos were transferred through three washes of chilled F-10 medium, in which the non-radioactive amino acids are present at 10- to 100-fold higher concentrations than the radioactive ones in the labeling medium. The embryos were then pooled appropriately in a 5 ml tube containing 0.25 ml of 0.25% alpha-amylase solution in 0.02 M sodium phosphate buffer pH 6.9 containing 0.006 M sodium chloride. After 1 h at room temperature, the embryos were solubilized by the addition of 0.25 ml of 2% sodium dodecyl sulfate and 10 M urea solution. Solubilization was complete within 30 min at room temperature. 0.5 ml of cold 20% trichloracetic acid (TCA) was then added to each tube and mixed thoroughly, and the samples placed in the cold for 2 h or overnight. The contents of each tube were then poured over a Whatman GF/A glass fiber filter 2.4 cm in diameter supported on a Millipore filtering apparatus. The filter was washed under gentle suction by rinsing first the lip of the tube with cold 5% TCA, then rinsing the entire tube with 6 5 ml aliquots of the same solution, each time pouring the rinse over the filter. No detectable radioactivity was found in selected sample tubes after this procedure, indicating that all radioactive material was quantitatively transferred to the filter. The filter and funnel were then washed with 15 ml of cold 5% TCA, 10 ml of hot 5% TCA (90°C), 5 ml of cold 5% TCA, and finally 10 ml of ether-ethanol (v/v). The filters were dried under an infra-red lamp, placed face up in glass scintillation vials, and covered with 10 ml of toluene-PPO-POPOP solution (5.0 g 2,5-diphenyloxazole, 0.1 g p-bis-2(5-phenyloxazolyl benzene)/l. Counting was performed in either a Beckman Model LS-133 or a Beckman Model LS-250 liquid scintillation counter, using the full spectrum window in the blue channel. Counting efficiency was determined to be 65% by using ^{14}C-*Chlorella* protein (New England Nuclear Corp.) as an internal standard. Background counts were determined separately for each group of embryos by exposing a comparable number of embryos of the same age to radioisotope under identical conditions, but in the presence of 100 μg/ml of puromycin (Nutritional Biochem.). This concentration was found in preliminary experiments to suppress incorporation in blastocysts by 96%. These background counts were subtracted from the appropriate experimental counts, so that the values presented represent only puromycin-sensitive incorporation.

Electrophoresis of embryonic protein

Embryos were prepared for electrophoresis by exposure to the radioisotope as described above. They were then washed briefly in normal saline, and pooled in 1 ml conical glass centrifuge tubes which had been siliconized. Large blastocysts were ruptured with a stainless steel wire and centrifuged at 5000 g for 10 min. The supernatant, considered to be almost pure blastocoelic fluid, was withdrawn and used for separate analysis. The cellular pellet was resuspended in 0.025 M phosphate buffer pH 7.0 containing 0.002 % Triton X-100 and frozen immediately. Early blastocyst and cleavage embryos were placed directly into the hypotonic buffer-detergent solution from the saline wash, and frozen. The embryos were thawed and refrozen three times in a dry ice-acetone bath, which was found by microscopic examination to disrupt more than 90 % of the cells. They were then centrifuged at 12,500 g for 20 min. If the thick mucin coats of the early embryos were not disrupted by this procedure, homogenization or sonication and repeat centrifugation were employed to liberate the soluble cellular protein. Sucrose was added to the final supernatant to a concentration of 5 %, and this solution was used as the protein sample for electrophoresis.

"Disc" electrophoresis of the embryonic protein was carried out in polyacrylamide gels measuring 2 × 60 mm. Gels were prepared at 7.5 % acrylamide pH 4.3 by the procedure of Reisfeld et al. [33] or at 5 % acrylamide pH 8.6 by the procedure of Clarke [8]. The gel column was overlaid with 3 mm of G-25 Superfine Sephadex presoaked in the appropriate buffer [23], and the sample solution layered over the Sephadex. Separation of the embryonic protein was carried out at 4° at a constant voltage of 100 volts for 90 min, when the tracking dye was 4–5 mm from the bottom of the gel. The gels were then stained with Ponceau-S for 5 min, and destained overnight in 5 % acetic acid. Protein bands containing between 0.1 and 0.5 μg of protein could be readily detected with this staining procedure.

After the visible bands had been located with respect to distance from the origin of migration, the gel was prepared for liquid scintillation counting by the method of Tishler and Epstein [39]. The gel was cut transversely into 1 mm sections, and each section placed in a separate glass scintillation vial and allowed to dry overnight. 0.1 ml of 30 % hydrogen peroxide was then added to each vial, and the vials were placed in a water bath at 50°C for 8 to 12 h, or until the gel was obviously in solution. After cooling, 1.0 ml of NCS reagent (Nuclear Chicago) and 10 ml of toluene-PPO-POPOP solution were added to each vial and the contents mixed thoroughly

by shaking. The vials were allowed to stand at least 24 h before counting, and each sample was counted a minimum of 3 times. Counting efficiency for ^{14}C was determined to be 74 %, and is stated by Tishler & Epstein [39] to be approx. 23 % for tritium in this system.

Unused culture medium containing radioisotope was subjected to electrophoresis as a control. Gels which had not been used for radioactive separations were sliced and used as background counts. The full spectrum counts in these non-radioactive gel slices varied between 78 and 96 CPM. The experimental values presented for the embryonic proteins are actual counts minus a standard 100 CPM.

RESULTS

The incorporation of radioisotope into TCA-insoluble material by the preimplantation rabbit embryo is shown at daily intervals throughout the preimplantation period in table 1. The results are expressed as CPM per embryo and, of perhaps greater relevance, as CPM per cell. The developmental event of interest in these experiments—the formation of the blastocyst—begins on the average late in the third day post coitum in the rabbit. Embryos obtained at exactly four days post coitum, even from the same doe, may be either late morulae or early blastocysts. These 4 day values are thus transitional ones with respect to this morphogenetic event.

The patterns of radioactivity obtained in the electrophoretic separations of labeled embryonic proteins are presented in figs 1, 2, and 3. These patterns were obtained from 88 2-day embryos applied to a single gel, 96 4-day embryos applied to duplicate gels, and 12 6-day embryos applied to triplicate gels, respectively. The reader's at-

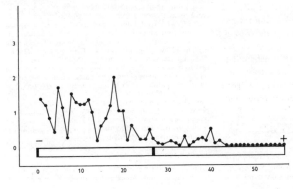

Fig. 1. Electrophoretic separation of ^3H-labeled proteins from 2 day rabbit embryos on polyacrylamide gel pH 8.6. Protein sample approx. 7 μg.

Table 1. *Incorporation of* ^{14}*C-amino acids by preimplantation rabbit embryos during a 4 h exposure to the radioisotope* in vitro

Embryo age (days post coitum) at time of exposure to radioisotope	No. of embryos used	Cell no. per embryo[a]	CPM per embryo	CPM per cell
Unfertilized ova	65	1	0	0
1	65	2	7	3.5
2	87	16	6	0.38
3	69	128	18	0.14
4	27	1,024	37	0.036
5	20	8,000	2,300	0.29
6	9	80,000	29,000	0.36

[a] See ref. 10.

tention is called to the fact that the counts in the 6-day gels are an order of magnitude higher than those in the other gels. The 2-day embryos were labeled with tritium in order to achieve higher specific protein activities.

The gel and its visible protein bands are shown diagrammatically below the radioactivity pattern for each stage of development. In the 2- and 4-day gels, only 2 bands were clearly visible, one near the origin and the other rapidly migrating. This forward band is seen to be the leading band in the 6-day gels. Since these 2 bands appear consistently in all the preimplantation stages ex-

amined, and represent protein species present in sufficient quantity to produce visible staining, these proteins will be referred to as the embryonic "bulk proteins".

The resolution of protein bands in six-day embryos was greater when electrophoresis was carried out in acid rather than in basic gels. Total recovery of applied radioactivity, however, was only 5%, as compared with 30% in the basic gels. The pattern obtained from acid gel electrophoresis of 6-day cellular protein, as well as that obtained from six-day blastocoelic fluid protein, is shown in fig. 4.

Electrophoretic separation of culture medium containing radioisotope, carried out in both acid and basic gels, resulted in background values for all gel segments with the exception of a small radioactive peak near the center of the heavy albumin band, presumably due to nonspecific adsorption of the radioisotope to the albumin.

DISCUSSION

The quantitative data on radioisotope incorporation in the preimplantation rabbit embryo show that during cleavage, when the embryonic cell number is increasing 500 to 1000-fold, the rate of incorporation per embryo increases a mere 5-fold. The incorporation rate viewed on a per cell basis shows a corresponding decrease throughout cleavage. By contrast, the rate of

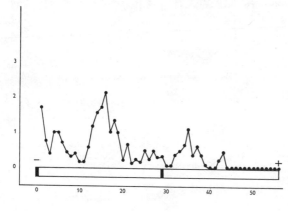

Fig. 2. Electrophoretic separation of ^{14}C-labeled proteins from 4 day rabbit embryos on polyacrylamide gels pH 8.6. Protein sample approx. 8 µg.

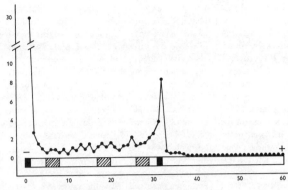

Fig. 3. Electrophoretic separation of ^{14}C-labeled cellular proteins from 6 day rabbit blastocysts on polyacrylamide gels pH 8.6. Protein sample approx. 12.5 μg.

incorporation per embryo increases directly with cell number in blastocysts (5- and 6-day embryos in table 1), and on a per cell basis is approximately equivalent to that found in the 2-day embryo.

Do these incorporation rates reflect normal protein synthetic rates, or might they be the result of variable intraembryonic precursor pools or altered permeability of embryonic membranes to exogenous amino acids? It has been amply demonstrated that both cleavage and blastocyst embryos of the rabbit require exogenous amino acids for in vitro development [13, 14], implying both that they are permeable to these molecules and that endogenous sources are insufficient at all stages to support growth. In a well-known study, Austin & Lovelock [2] have shown that the cleaving rabbit ovum is rapidly permeable to molecules with a molecular weight as high as 1200. Quantitative information on amino acid pools during preimplantation development of the rabbit is not available, but one might reasonably expect the radioisotope to be competing with a more formidable endogenous pool in blastocysts, considering the blastocoelic fluid as an integral part of the explanted embryo, than would be true in cleaving ova. Thus, incorporation values in blastocysts may be somewhat lowered by this endogenous pool, but these values are still remarkably high when compared

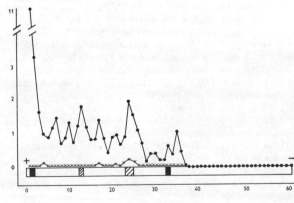

Fig. 4. Electrophoretic separations of ^{14}C-labeled cellular and blastocoelic fluid proteins from 6 day rabbit blastocysts on polyacrylamide gels pH 4.3. The cellular protein sample was approx. 10 μg, the blastocoelic fluid protein sample 90 μg. Both samples produced three identical bands; the band at 24 mm from the origin was absent in the blastocoelic fluid gel. ●—●, cell fraction; ×—×, blastocoelic fluid fraction.

Figs 1–4. Abscissa: Distance from origin (mm); *ordinate: figs 1, 2, 4,* cpm × 10⁻²; *fig. 3,* cpm × 10⁻³.

to cleaving stages. It has been found [14] that amino acid requirements for cleavage are somewhat variable, but the introduction of radioisotope by means of 15 different amino acids should nullify these temporary variations. It is proposed that the rates of incorporation given in table 1 are indeed true measures of the rate of protein synthesis, and that we may use the latter term without hesitation in discussing the data.

If replication of the embryonic genome during cleavage does not result in an increase in the rate of total embryonic protein synthesis, what hypotheses may be invoked to account for this phenomenon? Two hypotheses seem worthy of consideration. It will be seen in table 1 that there is no detectable synthesis occurring in the unfertilized rabbit ovum, and that immediately after fertilization there is marked synthetic activity. One hypothesis would have it, then, that the protein synthetic apparatus necessary to carry the embryo through cleavage is totally present in the zygote, and is merely parceled out to each blastomere with each cleavage division. This hypothesis would not allow for "utilization" of the embryonic genome for cleavage protein synthesis, and would be in accord with the situation found during cleavage in all non-mammalian systems which have been studied, i.e. it would include "stored" maternal messenger RNA as a corollary. The slight rise in synthetic rate per embryo up to four days post coitum could be accounted for by an increase in cell surface area during cleavage, resulting in a greater availability of the radioactive precursor.

A second hypothesis to account for the data is related to the "mass effect" seen in eukaryotic cells during the G2 period of the cell cycle. At this point in the cell cycle the genome has been replicated, yet the rate of protein synthesis does not double until after mitosis [20]. Whatever the factors are that suppress the "utilization" of the newly synthesized genetic material during the G2 period, these same factors may be operating in the rabbit embryo during cleavage. It will be recalled that cleavage does not result in overall embryonic growth; there is a progressive reduction in cell size, so that a morula of some 500 cells is no larger than the zygote. Thus, cleavage may not correspond precisely to "cell division" in the usual sense of producing progeny equal in size to the parent cell. This hypothesis would allow for transcription of the genome of the zygote, and during cleavage transcription would be limited to the genetic material of one, or at most a very few, of the blastomeres.

At least two facts militate against the second hypothesis. First, when reduction in cell size ceases at the end of cleavage and the embryo begins to grow as a blastocyst, the incorporation data show that the rate of protein synthesis per cell increases about 10-fold. Stated another way, each daughter cell, now the same size as the parent cell, becomes capable of synthesizing proteins 10 times more rapidly than its parent cell. It may be objected that the cells of the expanded blastocyst have much greater access to the radioisotope than do the cells of the tightly packed morula. This objection is countered by the second experimental fact: the rise in protein synthetic rate does not manifest itself fully until late in the fourth day post coitum, or several hours after the blastocyst is well-formed. Incorporation data from embryos at 4 days 19 h post coitum gave values of 570 cpm per embryo, or 0.14 cpm per cell. It is therefore apparent that the morphogenetic change does not confer an immediate advantage on the embryonic cells regarding their ability to incorporate radioisotope.

The data can, then, be interpreted in support of the first hypothesis, that the embryonic genome is not utilized for the protein synthesis which occurs during cleavage. Opposing this hypothesis is the sensitivity of the cleaving mouse [28, 38] and rabbit [26] embryo to actinomycin D. Cleavage of both species is inhibited by low concentrations of the antibiotic (10^{-8} to 10^{-9} M), levels which were found by Perry [32] to suppress nucleolar labeling selectively in cultured mammalian cells. This sensitivity of cleaving ova would suggest that ribosomal RNA synthesis is required for cleavage, and indeed Mintz [28] has shown nucleolar labeling as early as the 4-cell stage in mouse development. Comparable information is not yet available to define the onset of ribosomal RNA synthesis in the rabbit embryo. However, it might be pointed out that the t^{12}/t^{12} lethal mouse mutant, whose one striking abnormality is its deficiency in RNA synthesis, nevertheless does cleave normally [29]. And it remains to be proved that the actinomycin D is exerting its inhibitory effect on cleavage by means of its interference with DNA-dependent RNA synthesis, and not by means of one of its numerous "side effects" [22, 25, 31, 34, 35]. The point is not whether RNA synthesis occurs during cleavage of the mammalian embryo, since it quite evidently does. The point is rather whether sensitivity to actinomycin D unequivocally demonstrates that this RNA synthesis is *required* for cleavage, contrary to what has been found in non-mammalian systems [7, 19, 40]. It is entirely conceivable that RNA synthesis during cleavage is a preliminary to later normal development, in accord with these non-mammalian systems [18], and that the "side effects" of actinomycin D may be simply more damaging to the mammalian embryo than to the echinoderm or amphibian.

The electrophoretic data presented in figs 1, 2, and 3 answer the qualitative question regarding the increase in protein synthetic rate with blastocyst formation. The proteins synthesized by the blastocyst are not identical to those synthesized by cleaving embryos. The pattern of incorporation of radioisotope into soluble protein changes during the preimplantation period of rabbit development, a result which is not surprising. It is, perhaps, not altogether expected that the very early blastocyst, represented by the 4-day pattern, resembles the cleaving embryo more than it resembles a "mature" 6-day blastocyst in its synthetic pattern. The 2 bands which we have termed the embryonic "bulk" proteins do not account for any significant incorporation during cleavage and early blastocyst development, but show high incorporation in the 6-day blastocyst. This change in the pattern of incorporation has been described as one from "low coincidence with the bulk pattern to high coincidence" [17], and the same general pattern change has been found in the proteins synthesized during early

sea urchin embryogenesis [17, 36]. This change in the rabbit embryo is clearly associated with the onset of true growth, and the requirement for the synthesis of new bulk proteins at this time, whatever they may be, is obvious.

In fig. 4 it can be seen that the specific activity of the blastocoelic fluid is negligible when compared to that of the cellular proteins of the 6-day blastocyst. This finding suggests either that the newly-synthesized cellular proteins find their way into the blastocyst cavity relatively slowly, or that the blastocoelic proteins are derived from the uterine fluids rather than from the embryo. It has been shown that "blastokinin", a specific protein found in rabbit uterine fluids and synthesized outside the embryo, nevertheless comprises about 35 % of the blastocoelic fluid protein [24]. It appears likely, in view of other studies on the transfer of maternal proteins to the embryo [3, 16], that the majority of blastocoelic proteins are derived from the uterine environment.

The data presented here demonstrate that the transformation of the rabbit morula into a blastocyst is associated with a tenfold increase in the rate of protein synthesis per cell, and that the synthesis of embryonic bulk proteins is significantly detectable only in the blastocyst. These data are consistent with the notion that protein synthesis during cleavage is occurring in the absence of direct genomic control, and that cell division in the blastocyst is accompanied by replication of the rate-limiting factor or factors which govern protein synthesis. Since there is a qualitative change in protein synthesis with the formation of the blastocyst, it is proposed that the rate-limiting factor is genetic expression. At which "level" genetic expression is occurring cannot be determined from these experiments. It may be that messengers for this new protein synthesis are being transcribed throughout cleavage, but not translated until the blastocyst phase of development [18]. Terman and Gross [37] have demonstrated changing patterns of protein synthesis in developing sea urchin embryos maintained in the presence of actinomycin D, and suggest that translation level control of protein synthesis may be a rather general phenomenon in higher organisms. Further work is obviously needed to clarify this situation in the developing rabbit embryo.

A final point should be made. The increase in protein synthetic rate occurs after the morphogenetic changes resulting in the formation of a blastocyst are well underway. Other metabolic parameters which have been investigated, such as oxygen consumption [15] and the utilization of single carbon energy sources [12], likewise show changes late in the fourth day post coitum. It would appear either that the initiation of this morphogenetic event does not require direct genetic intervention, or that it is quantitatively undetectable by the methods used here but qualitatively highly important for development. When the mechanism of cavitation is better understood, it may then be possible to decide which of these two alternatives is correct.

The work was supported by US Atomic Energy Commission contract no. AT (11-1)-1957. One of us (C. M.) was the recipient of postdoctoral fellowship no. 5 F2 HD-32,206-02 from the National Institute of Child Health and Human Development, USPHS, during a portion of this work.

REFERENCES

1. Adams, C E, J endocrinol 16 (1958) 283.
2. Austin, C R & Lovelock, J E, Exptl cell res 15 (1958) 260.
3. Brambell, W F R, Hemmings, W A & Henderson, M, Antibodies and embryos. Athlone Press, London (1951).
4. Brinster, R L, Exptl cell res 32 (1963) 205.
5. — J exptl zool 158 (1965) 59.
6. — Ibid. 158 (1965) 69.
7. Brown, D D & Gurdon, J B, Proc natl acad sci US 51 (1964) 139.
8. Clarke, J T, Ann N Y acad sci 121 (1965) 428.
9. Daniel, J C, Jr, Am zool 3 (1963) 526.
10. — Am naturalist 98 (1964) 85.
11. — J embryol exptl morphol 13 (1965) 83.
12. — Exptl cell res 47 (1967) 619.
13. Daniel, J C, Jr & Krishnan, R S, J cell physiol 70 (1967) 155.
14. Daniel, J C, Jr & Olson, J D, J reprod fertil 15 (1968) 453.
15. Fridhandler, L, Exptl cell res 22 (1961) 303.
16. Glass, L E, Am zool 3 (1963) 135.
17. Gross, P R, Current topics in developmental biology (ed A Monroy & A A Moscona) p. 1. Academic Press, New York (1967).
18. — New Engl j med 276 (1967) 1239.
19. Gross, P R, Malkin, L I & Moyer, W A, Proc natl acad sci US 51 (1964) 407.
20. Halvorson, H O, Bock, R M, Tauro, P, Epstein, R & LaBerge, M, Cell synchrony (ed I L Cameron & G M Padilla) p. 102. Academic Press, New York (1966).
21. Ham, R G, Exptl cell res 29 (1963) 515.
22. Honig, G R & Rabinovitz, M, Science 149 (1965) 1504.
23. Hydén, H, Bjurstam, K & McEwen, B, Anal biochem 17 (1966) 1.
24. Krishnan, R S & Daniel, J C, Jr, Science 158 (1967) 490.
25. Laszlo, J, Miller, D S, McCarty, K S & Hochstein, P, Science 151 (1966) 1007.
26. Manes, C. In preparation.
27. Mans, R J & Novelli, G D, Arch biochem 94 (1961) 48.
28. Mintz, B, J exptl zool 157 (1964) 85.
29. — Ibid. 157 (1964) 267.
30. Monesi, V & Salfi, V, Exptl cell res 46 (1967) 632.
31. Pastan, I & Friedman, R M, Science 160 (1968) 316.
32. Perry, R P, Exptl cell res 29 (1963) 400.
33. Reisfeld, R A, Lewis, V J & Williams, D E, Nature 195 (1962) 281.
34. Revel, M, Hiatt, H H & Revel, J-P, Science 146 (1964) 1311.
35. Soeiro, R & Amos, H, Biochim biophys acta 129 (1966) 406.
36. Spiegel, M, Ozaki, H & Tyler, A, Biochem biophys res commun 21 (1965) 135.
37. Terman, S A & Gross, P R, Biochem biophys res commun 21 (1965) 595.
38. Thomson, J L & Biggers, J D, Exptl cell res 41 (1966) 411.
39. Tishler, P V & Epstein, C J, Anal biochem 22 (1968) 89.
40. Wilt, F H, Develop biol 9 (1964) 299.

AUTHOR INDEX

KEY-WORD TITLE INDEX